Key Topics in
Human Diseases for Dental Students

The KEY TOPICS Series

Advisors:

TM Craft *Department of Anaesthesia and Intensive Care, Royal United Hospital, Bath, UK*
CS Garrard *Intensive Therapy Unit, John Radcliffe Hospital, Oxford, UK*
PM Upton *Department of Anaesthesia, Royal Cornwall Hospital, Treliske, Truro, UK*

Accident and Emergency Medicine, Second Edition
Anaesthesia; Clinical Aspects, Third Edition
Cardiac Surgery
Cardiovascular Medicine
Chronic Pain, Second Edition
Critical Care
Evidence-Based Medicine
Gastroenterology
General Surgery
Neonatology, Second Edition
Neurology
Obstetrics and Gynaecology, Second Edition
Oncology
Ophthalmology, Second Edition
Oral and Maxillofacial Surgery
Orthopaedic Surgery
Orthopaedic Trauma Surgery
Otolaryngology, Second Edition
Paediatrics, Second Edition
Psychiatry
Renal Medicine
Respiratory Medicine
Thoracic Surgery
Trauma

Forthcoming titles include:

Critical Care, Second Edition
Plastic and Reconstructive Surgery
Sexual Health

Key Topics in
Human Diseases for Dental Students

Prasanna Sooriakumaran
BMedSci(Hons) BMBS(Hons) MRCS(Eng)
Clinical Lecturer in Prostate Cancer, University of Surrey & Special Study Modules Tutor, Guy's, King's & St. Thomas' School of Medicine, Dentistry, and Biomedical Sciences, King's College London

Channa Jayasena
MA MB BChir MRCP
Specialist Registrar, Division of Endocrinology and Metabolism, The Hammersmith Hospital, London

Crispian Scully
CBE MD PhD MDS MRCS FDSRCS FDSRCPS FFDRCSI FDSRCSE FRCPath FMedSci
Dean and Director of Studies and Research, Eastman Dental Institute for Oral Health Sciences, and International Centres for Excellence in Dentistry, University College London

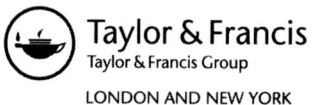
Taylor & Francis
Taylor & Francis Group

LONDON AND NEW YORK

© 2005 Taylor & Francis, an imprint of the Taylor & Francis Group

First published in the United Kingdom in 2005 by Taylor & Francis, an imprint of the Taylor & Francis Group, 2 Park Square, Milton Park, Abingdon, Oxon OX14 4RN

Tel.:   +44 (0) 20 7017 6000
Fax.:   +44 (0) 20 7017 6699
E-mail: info.medicine@tandf.co.uk
Website: http://www.tandf.co.uk/medicine

Important Note from the Publisher
The information contained within this book was obtained by Taylor & Francis from sources believed by us to be reliable. However, while every effort has been made to ensure its accuracy, no responsibility for loss or injury whatsoever occasioned to any person acting or refraining from action as a result of information contained herein can be accepted by the authors or publishers.

The reader should remember that medicine is a constantly evolving science and while the authors and publishers have ensured that all dosages, applications and practices are based on current indications, there may be specific practices which differ between communities. You should always follow the guidelines laid down by the manufacturers of specific products and the relevant authorities in the country in which you are practising.

A CIP record for this book is available from the British Library.

Library of Congress Cataloging-in-Publication Data

Data available on application

ISBN 1 84184 435 7

Distributed in North and South America by
Taylor & Francis
2000 NW Corporate Blvd
Boca Raton, FL 33431, USA

Within Continental USA
Tel.: 800 272 7737; Fax.: 800 374 3401
Outside Continental USA
Tel.: 561 994 0555; Fax.: 561 361 6018
E-mail: orders@crcpress.com

Distributed in the rest of the world by
Thomson Publishing Services
Cheriton House
North Way
Andover, Hampshire SP10 5BE, UK
Tel.: +44 (0)1264 332424
E-mail: salesorder.tandf@thomsonpublishingservices.co.uk

Composition by Scribe Design Ltd, Ashford, Kent, UK

Printed and bound in Great Britain by TJ International Ltd, Padstow, Cornwall

Contents

About the Authors

Prasanna Sooriakumaran graduated with honours from the University of Nottingham and is currently a PhD student and a Special Study Modules Tutor at GKT Medical School, King's College London. He has taught dental, medical, physiotherapy, neuroscience and human biology students at undergraduate level, both at the University of Nottingham and at schools in the University of London.

Channa Jayasena graduated from the University of Cambridge and is currently working in Endocrinology at Hammersmith Hospital, London. He has had teaching commitments at the University of Cambridge and is currently a BSc supervisor for medical students at Imperial College London.

Professor Crispian Scully CBE is Dean of the Eastman Dental Institute, University College London. He has written over 650 papers and 30 books in dentistry and medicine, and has many years of teaching experience of undergraduate dental and medical students in several universities in the UK and abroad.

Dedication

This book is dedicated to Sumi, Dilan, Zoe and Frances

Preface

The main aim of this book is to aid clinical dental students to gain a sound, broad understanding of the main medical and surgical conditions they may encounter, both in their undergraduate examinations and their professional practice. In a book of this size and nature, it is impossible to be comprehensive and we have made no attempt at this. Rather, we have tried to condense the essence of the chosen topics into 'bitesize' chunks for the dental reader so that the most important elements of the condition, together with any specific dental relevance, are covered. The 'Five facts' summary boxes are there to give the 'take home' messages for each chapter and serve as an aide-mémoire.

We do not envisage this book replacing that of standard, larger textbooks, but have found from our own experiences that dental students need a revision-style guide through the wide breadth of medical and surgical diseases. We also envisage that this book will be of use to medical and other health professionals as a quick revision guide.

P Sooriakumaran, C Jayasena, C Scully
London, 2005

Acknowledgements

We would like to thank our own clinical teachers, past and present, for their words of wisdom in the preparation of this book. We are grateful to the staff at Taylor & Francis, in particular Mr Robert Peden and Ms Teresa Netzler, for their continued support.

Most of all, we would like to thank the numerous dental students, especially those at the dental schools in the University of London, for providing the inspiration for this work.

Abdominal aortic aneurysms

An aneurysm is an abnormal dilatation of a vessel. The incidence of abdominal aortic aneurysms (AAA) increases with age: they are common in older men and can often be fatal. AAA are said to arise as a consequence of arteries becoming stiffer, wider, longer and, most importantly, calcified. This can lead to dilatation in the arteries; once the artery is >150% of its normal diameter, it is said to be aneurysmal. The stiffness can be attributed to the build up of atheromatous plaques due to hyperlipidaemia.

AAA may be due to a gene mutation in one of the structural proteins of connective tissue but the main other risk factors are hypertension, hyperlipidaemia, ischaemic heart disease, and peripheral vascular disease. Smoking has also been implicated in the development of AAA because free radicals damage major blood vessels.

Clinical features

Many patients with AAA are asymptomatic and the aneurysm is diagnosed incidentally during clinical examination (pulsatile, expansile, epigastric mass on abdominal examination) or imaging – computed tomography (CT) or ultrasound of the abdomen – for other reasons. Symptomatic AAA may present with epigastric pain, back pain, malaise or weight loss, or there may be rupture – a serious emergency.

Patients with ruptured AAA present with:

- severe central abdominal pain
- hypovolaemic shock.

It is important to recognize ruptured AAA as this is a true surgical emergency. Due to the high rate of morbidity and mortality associated with ruptured AAA, accurate diagnosis is necessary before rupture. Helical CT and CT angiography are becoming available, and have certain advantages over conventional CT and ultrasound for diagnosis, such as better 3D visualization.

Management

Indications for AAA surgery include:

- ruptured AAA (surgical emergency)
- symptomatic AAA (as this may indicate the AAA is more likely to rupture)
- size of asymptomatic AAA > 5.5 cm (as this may indicate the AAA is more likely to rupture).

Elective surgical repair of AAA has a mortality of ~5%. Ruptured AAA has a mortality of >70%, dropping to ~50% if the patient survives until he reaches hospital. Hence it is important to do surgical repair in the elective situation rather than as an emergency procedure.

Surgical repairs of aneurysms were first done by open laparotomy (midline incision from the xiphisternum to the pubis). During open surgery the aneurysm is opened longitudinally and cleared of its contents, and a graft placed to bridge the gap and form an anastomosis.

Endovascular repair involves radiographically guided intraluminal placement of a prosthetic graft on a wire mesh into the abdominal aorta via a small groin incision, thus avoiding the morbidity and mortality associated with major open abdominal surgery. If grafting is deemed unsuitable, stents can be placed instead.

Complications

The most important complication of AAA is that it can result in fatality from haemorrhagic shock, cardiac arrest and multi-system organ failure. Ischaemia to the spinal cord can cause paraplegia.

Screening

Ultrasonography is the standard method of screening and monitoring non-ruptured AAA. However CT and CT angiography are now replacing this. It is estimated that a single ultrasound at 65 years could reduce deaths from AAA rupture by 70% in a screened population but screening at present is reserved for high-risk groups, such as those with a positive family history and hypertensive smokers.

All AAA <5.5 cm should be monitored closely with annual ultrasound or CT. In high-risk cases, such as women, those with connective tissue disease (e.g. Marfan's syndrome) and those with other comorbidities, surgery may be considered early.

Five facts

1. AAA is not uncommon in the elderly.
2. AAA is a disease of arteriopaths.
3. Ruptured AAA is a true surgical emergency.
4. AAA >5.5 cm should be repaired electively in most circumstances.
5. Small AAA should be monitored regularly (6–12 monthly) with abdominal ultrasound or CT.

Acute abdominal pain

Features of pain

Every student should be able to elicit a history asking about the salient features of pain:

- **site**
- **character (e.g. sharp, stabbing, colicky, dull, aching, tightness)**
- time and nature of onset
- severity (e.g. marks out of 10)
- progression
- duration
- radiation
- precipitating/aggravating factors
- relieving factors (including analgesia).

The two most useful features to make the diagnosis in the majority of cases are the site and character.

We will now discuss various abdominal pathologies and relate them to the above features, emphasizing site and character.

Peptic ulcer disease (PUD)

Peptic ulcers are usually either duodenal (DU) or gastric (GU), although they can occur in the oesophagus or within a Meckel's diverticulum. The normal stomach secretes acid and pepsin and has a mucosal barrier to protect it from these substances. When the mucosal barrier is compromised, the acid and pepsin cause mucosal ulceration. The oesophagus and Meckel's diverticulum have no protective mucosal barrier and thus can also ulcerate if acid is in contact with them.

The usual cause for the barrier failure is infection with the spiral-shaped, Gram-negative bacillus (rod), *Helicobacter pylori*. In rare cases patients with PUD have Zollinger–Ellison syndrome (named after two Ohio surgeons) in which an islet cell tumour of the pancreas produces a gastrin-like substance.

Risk factors
- Middle-aged and elderly people with other risk factors.
- Non-steroidal anti-inflammatory drugs (NSAIDs).
- Corticosteroids.
- Alcohol.
- Smoking.
- Asian ethnic origin.
- Social class 1 (? stress-related).
- Head injury (Cushing's ulcer).
- Severe burns (Curling's ulcer).

Symptoms
- Typically, epigastric pain.
- Heartburn or indigestion.
- Acid/water brash.

However, there are differences between DU and GU (Table 1).

Table 1 Differences between duodenal (DU) and gastric (GU) ulcers

Feature	DU	GU
Site	Epigastric	Epigastric
Onset	2–3 hours after eating	Soon after eating
Severity	Variable	Variable
Character	Burning sensation	Burning sensation
Progression	4–6 month cycle	Comes and goes in a 2–3 month cycle
Duration	1–2 months	Few weeks
Precipitating factors	Stress	Eating, especially spicy foods
Relieving factors	Eating	Vomiting
Radiation	None or to the back	None or to the back

Special investigations
- Faecal occult bloods (may show blood in the stools – although the specificity and sensitivity of this investigation is poor).
- Oesophagogastroduodenoscopy (OGD) to visualize the ulcer directly and take biopsy.
- OGD-directed biopsy is more important if the ulcer is gastric, as many of these ulcers may be malignant, and naked eye inspection is not accurate at differentiating benign from malignant GUs.
- *H. pylori* detection:
    - 'clo' test – this works on the principle that *H. pylori* is a urease-containing bacterium that splits urea into ammonia, which is of a different pH. Hence, if the biopsy material causes this change of pH when added to a solution of urea, then *H. pylori* is present.
    - Breath test.
    - Antibody test.
    The clo test is the only one of the above three tests that is in routine clinical use.
- Barium meal has been superseded by OGD.

Management
- Medical
    - Eradicate *H. pylori* with triple therapy: metronidazole, amoxicillin, and omeprazole.
    - Reduce acid secretion, by using proton pump inhibitors (PPIs) such as omeprazole or pantoprazole. Histamine H2-receptor antagonists are no longer used as first-line treatment.

It is vital to re-OGD all GUs after 6 weeks of medical treatment to re-exclude malignancy.
- Surgical
  - This is reserved nowadays for unresponsive cases where various types of gastrectomy may be performed, or for the complications of PUD.

Complications of PU
- Bleeding.
- Perforation.

Any patient suspected of having these complications warrants immediate assessment by a surgeon; both conditions are indications for emergency surgery by open laparotomy. A bleeding PU presents with upper gastrointestinal bleeding (see chapter on gastrointestinal bleeding), whereas a perforated PU presents with peritonitis (inflammation of the peritoneum; often fatal).

Signs of peritonitis
- Extreme pain, aggravated by movement.
- Fever.
- Cold, sweaty skin.
- Rapid, shallow breathing.
- Patient looks very ill.
- Rigid, silent abdomen.
- Shock is a late sign.
- Air under the diaphragm is a classical feature on an erect chest X-ray (seen in 70% of patients with perforated PU).
- Death occurs in up to 10% of cases, most often due to delay in time to surgery.

Acute pancreatitis

In acute pancreatitis, activated pancreatic enzymes (e.g. trypsin, chymotrypsin) leak into the substance of the pancreas and cause autodigestion of the gland. Obstruction of the pancreatic duct would cause this (e.g. from a gallstone) but there are other causes:

- **Gallstones**
- **Ethanol (alcohol)**
- Trauma
- Steroids
- Mumps and other viruses
- Autoimmune disorders
- Scorpion bites (!)
- Hyperlipidaemia
- ERCP (endoscopic retrograde cholangiopancreatography)
- Drugs.

These causes can be easily committed to memory if the student remembers what he/she might typically do on a Saturday night ('GET SMASHED').

Gallstones or alcohol are the causes in >80% of cases.

Pancreatitis can vary in severity from a very mild inflammation to a severe, necrotizing inflammation with massive destruction of the gland.

Clinical features

The clinical features of acute pancreatitis are given in Table 2.

Table 2 Clinical features of acute pancreatitis

Pain	Acute pancreatitis
Site	Epigastric
Onset	Sudden
Severity	Variable
Character	Gnawing
Progression	Gets worse gradually
Duration	Variable
Precipitating factors	Alcoholic binge
Relieving factors	Opiate analgesia
Radiation	To the back

Acute pancreatitis is also often associated with frequent bouts of vomiting and nausea.

Investigations

Due to the damaged pancreas, amylase gets released into the circulation and hence the serum amylase level is typically grossly raised (>10 times normal).

Management

Management can vary from simple rest (nasogastric tube, nil by mouth, and intravenous fluids – 'drip and suck') to intensive care in ITU, depending on the severity of the disease. Surgery is reserved for haemorrhagic, necrotizing pancreatitis to remove any necrotic pancreatic tissue. The role of antibiotics remains controversial.

Acute appendicitis

Acute appendicitis is one of the most common causes of acute abdominal pain. Chances are the reader will have suffered from, or know someone who has suffered from, appendicitis. In most cases, the appendix lumen gets obstructed by a faecolith, causing the inflammation. Occasionally, especially in the elderly, a carcinoma of the caecum may cause the obstruction, and appendicitis is then the presenting feature of this more significant pathology.

Clinical features

The clinical features of appendicitis are given in Table 3.

Table 3 Clinical features of appendicitis

Pain	Appendicitis
Site	Starts central, and then moves to right iliac fossa (RIF)
Onset	Gradual over 2–3 days
Severity	Variable
Character	Starts vague but becomes more sharp
Progression	Constant
Duration	Few days
Precipitating factors	None specific
Relieving factors	Analgesia
Radiation	Central to RIF

The diagnosis of appendicitis is often extremely difficult, and various scoring systems have been developed. The only one of any clinical use is the modified Alvarado (or MANTREL) score:

- Migrating right iliac fossa (RIF) pain
- Anorexia
- Nausea/vomiting
- Tender RIF
- Rebound tenderness
- Elevated temperature >37.5°C
- Leukocytosis.

The greater the number of above features present, the greater the likelihood that the patient has acute appendicitis. However, a study by the first author (P.S.) has shown that clinical judgement is still better than this scoring system in patients presenting to an emergency department.

Investigations
Apart from routine blood tests – e.g. full blood count (FBC) may show a raised white blood cell count (WBC) and C-reactive protein (CRP) – there is no consensus regarding the use of abdominal ultrasound or diagnostic laparoscopy.

Management
Some surgeons prefer to proceed directly to appendicectomy, while others perform laparoscopy to exclude gynaecological causes in females (e.g. acute salpingitis) and proceed to laparoscopic appendicectomy if the appendix looks inflamed. It is important to try and perform an appendicectomy before the appendix perforates, as this will result in the patient being much sicker and making the operation more difficult.

Bowel obstruction

Both the small bowel and the large bowel can become obstructed by mechanical causes and cause pain. Small bowel obstruction (SBO) is typically due to either adhesions from previous surgery (managed conservatively with 'drip and suck') or to a hernia (see chapter on hernias). Large bowel obstruction (LBO) is more sinister, with the commonest cause being an obstructing colorectal carcinoma (see chapter on colorectal cancer). Hence, LBO is usually managed with emergency laparotomy, with resection of the cancer and the formation of a diverting colostomy.

There are four cardinal symptoms and signs of bowel obstruction:

- colicky abdominal pain
- vomiting
- abdominal distension
- absolute constipation (i.e. no faeces or flatus passed).

Bowel obstruction can usually be diagnosed on plain abdominal X-ray, where dilated loops of bowel proximal to the obstruction can be seen. Small bowel loops tend to be more centrally placed than large bowel loops. Large bowel also has haustrations (lines that go only part of the way across the lumen on X-ray) as compared to the valvulae coniventes of small bowel (lines that go all the way across the lumen). These X-ray features distinguish SBO from LBO.

Irritable bowel syndrome (IBS)

IBS is a common functional disorder of the gastrointestinal smooth muscle that affects roughly 10% of adults in the UK. It is characterized by abdominal pain or discomfort that is associated with a change in bowel habit, and is relieved by defaecation. Attacks are typically precipitated by certain foods, often oily or spicy preparations. Management is with reassurance, anti-spasmodic drugs and dietary manipulation.

IBS is a diagnosis of exclusion, and students should not make this diagnosis without full gastrointestinal evaluation.

Other causes of acute abdominal pain

The following list is not exhaustive, but covers the main other differential diagnoses. All the following conditions have been covered in other chapters of this book:

- acute cholecystitis
- biliary colic
- ureteric colic
- diverticular disease
- inflammatory bowel disease
- abdominal aortic aneurysm
- myocardial infarction
- diabetic ketoacidosis
- pneumonia.

Reference

1. A Comparison of Clinical Judgment of Accident and Emergency Doctors and the Modified Alvarado Score in Evaluating the Need for Surgical Referral in Cases of Suspected Acute Appendicitis: Sooriakumaran P, Dovell D, Brown R. Int J Surg (2005) In press.

Five facts

1. Pain should be described in terms of its site, onset, severity, character, progression, duration, precipitating and relieving factors, and radiation.
2. Appendicitis is the most common cause of an acute abdomen.
3. Peptic ulcers are more common with stress and smoking.
4. Gastric ulcers may be malignant and should always be biopsied.
5. Acute pancreatitis is commonly caused by gallstones or alcohol.

Adrenal disorders

- The adrenal medulla develops embryologically as part of the sympathetic nervous system and secretes catecholamines such as noradrenaline (norepinephrine) and adrenaline (epinephrine) to promote peripheral vasoconstriction, tachycardia and increased myocardial contractility.
- The adrenal cortex secretes:
  1. *Glucocorticoids* such as cortisol that are released in response to stimulation by adrenocorticotrophic hormone (ACTH) from the anterior part of the pituitary gland. Corticosteroids are an essential part of the body's response to stressors such as trauma, infection, general anaesthesia, surgery, pain, stress, fever, burns and hypoglycaemia.
  2. *Mineralocorticoids* such as aldosterone that are released in response to stimulation from renin/angiotensin and the sympathetic nervous system. They act on the kidney to promote salt and water retention, and increase potassium and acid (hydrogen) secretion. Renin, an enzyme that converts angiotensinogen to angiotensin 1, is produced by the renal juxtaglomerular apparatus, in response to low serum sodium or renal perfusion. Angiotensin I is converted by angiotensin-converting enzyme in the lung parenchyma, to the active angiotensin II, which stimulates aldosterone release.
  3. *Androgens*, e.g. DHEA (dehydroepiandrosterone), are important in the production of secondary sexual characteristics such as pubic hair, the pubertal growth spurt and the lowering of the male voice after puberty.
- Disorders of the adrenal gland may cause either hypofunction (Addison's disease) or hyperfunction of hormone secretion. Adrenocortical hyperfunction may lead to release of excessive:
  - glucocorticoids (Cushing's syndrome)
  - mineralocorticoids (Conn's syndrome or hyperaldosteronism)
  - androgens (congenital adrenal hyperplasia).

Addison's disease

Addison's disease (primary adrenal insufficiency) is caused by inadequate secretion of cortisol and/or aldosterone from the adrenal glands.

Aetiology
Addison's disease is most commonly an autoimmune condition. Other causes include:

- tuberculosis (TB)
- neoplasms such as metastatic carcinoma or lymphoma
- haemorrhage associated with meningococcal septicaemia (Waterhouse–Friderichsen syndrome)
- amyloidosis
- systemic fungal infections (eg. histoplasmosis).

Clinical features
Patients often complain of tiredness, dizziness, nausea and vomiting. Clinical signs may include hypotension and hypoglycaemia. Brown or black pigmentation of the

oral mucosa is seen in over 75% of patients with Addison's disease. Hyper-pigmentation is related to high levels of melanocyte-stimulating hormone (MSH) and particularly affects areas normally pigmented or exposed to trauma.

Investigations
In Addison's disease, basal 9 am plasma cortisol levels are low and there is an inade-quate rise in cortisol levels 30 and 60 min after injection of Synacthen (tetracosac-tide), a synthetic ACTH analogue.

Serum sodium and bicarbonate are low; serum potassium is high.

Treatment
Acute adrenal insufficiency is managed as follows:

- lay the patient flat with the legs raised
- give hydrocortisone (100–200 mg) intravenously
- summon medical assistance.

Chronically, Addison's disease is treated with oral hydrocortisone (cortisol) replace-ment.

Cushing's syndrome

Cushing's syndrome is defined as an excess of glucocorticoids as a result of one of three main mechanisms:

1. *ACTH-secreting pituitary adenoma.* This is termed *Cushing's disease.* Excess ACTH stimulates cortisol secretion from the adrenals and also stimulates melanin produc-tion, causing increased skin pigmentation. Both ACTH and cortisol levels are high.
2. *Ectopic ACTH secretion.* Certain malignant neoplasms (particularly small-cell bronchial carcinoma) may secrete ACTH.
3. *Adrenal adenoma.* This benign neoplasm results in overproduction of cortisol. ACTH secretion is low due to negative feedback by cortisol.

Clinical features
Excess glucocorticoids lead to classical *cushingoid* features, which are:

- Fat redistribution, leading to a *moon face* and *buffalo hump* on the neck. It also leads to *centripetal fat distribution*, i.e. increased fat on the thorax and abdomen, with less fat on the legs and arms.
- *Proximal myopathy*: wasting of muscles of thighs and upper arms.
- *Acne*, due to stimulation of sebaceous gland activity.
- *Abdominal striae, thin skin, skin bruising* and *poor wound healing*, due to the catabolic state induced by cortisol.
- *Hirsutism* (excess body hair).
- *Hypertension*, due to mild mineralocorticoid effect on the kidneys, and sympa-thetic stimulation.
- *Osteoporosis*.
- *Insulin resistance and gluconeogenesis*, which may lead to *diabetes mellitus*.
- *Peptic ulceration*.
- *Psychiatric conditions*, e.g. euphoria, psychosis.

Investigations
Investigations are initially directed at establishing the diagnosis and then of distinguishing which of the three mechanisms is responsible for the excess cortisol.
    Diagnosis of Cushing's syndrome is by:

- *24-hour urinary secretion of cortisol*: increased.
- *Low-dose dexamethasone suppression test* (dexamethasone 0.5 mg is given every 6 hours for 48 hours): failure of cortisol levels to drop at the end of the test.

Distinguishing the cause of Cushing's syndrome is by:

- *Plasma ACTH* measurement: if it is very low, then the diagnosis is of adrenal adenoma (with suppression of ACTH via negative feedback). If ACTH is raised, then a *high-dose dexamethasone suppression test* is performed.
- *High-dose dexamethasone suppression test* (2 mg dexamethasone every 6 hours for 48 hours). A failure in the suppression of cortisol suggests ectopic ACTH secretion from a tumour. Suppression of cortisol suggests a pituitary adenoma.

Further investigations
- Loss of diurnal rhythm of serum cortisol: cortisol levels are highest at 9 a.m., and lowest at midnight. In Cushing's syndrome, this pattern is lost.
- Urea and electrolytes: the mineralocorticoid effect of cortisol may produce hypokalaemia and a metabolic alkalosis (raised bicarbonate).
- Scans: a magnetic resonance imaging (MRI) scan may detect a pituitary adenoma; a computed tomography (CT) scan may detect an adrenal adenoma or bronchial carcinoma.

Treatment
Resection of the underlying adrenal or pituitary adenoma leads to cure of Cushing's syndrome. ACTH-secreting tumours tend to be metastatic, and are therefore not amenable to resection. In this situation, drugs which inhibit the synthesis of glucocorticoids, such as ketoconazole and metyrapone, may be used.

Dental aspects
Patients, once treated, are maintained on corticosteroid replacement therapy and are then at risk from an adrenal crisis if subjected to operation, anaesthesia or trauma.

Conn's syndrome

Conn's syndrome is characterized by excess secretion of mineralocorticoids, caused by an aldosterone-secreting adrenal cortex tumour. Affected individuals are asymptomatic, and have no abnormal clinical signs except hypertension.
    Urea and electrolytes demonstrate a hypokalaemic metabolic alkalosis.
    Lying and standing serum renin/aldosterone measurements: aldosterone levels are raised and the level of renin is suppressed. A CT scan is used to localize the adrenal adenoma.
    Spironolactone is an aldosterone receptor antagonist which may be used to directly inhibit its effects. Surgical resection of the tumour provides definitive treatment.

Dental aspects
If bilateral adrenalectomy has been carried out, the patient is at risk from collapse during dental treatment and therefore requires corticosteroid cover.

Congenital adrenal hyperplasia

Congenital adrenal hyperplasia (CAH) is due to genetic deficiency in adrenal enzymes such as 11β-hydroxylase or 17-hydroxylase, leading to excess androgens. This leads to virilization of females (e.g. clitoromegaly and male pattern of pubic hair) and precocious puberty.

Phaeochromocytoma

Phaeochromocytoma is a rare neoplasm of the adrenal medulla which secretes excess catecholamines. Clinical features occur due to increased levels of catecholamines – paroxysmal attacks of anxiety, palpitations, sweating, tachycardia and hypertension.

Diagnosis is by demonstration of high levels of catecholamines (e.g. noradrenaline) or metabolites of catecholamines (e.g. vanillylmandelic acid (VMA)) in a 24-hour urine collection. CT scan will show the enlarged adrenal gland. Phenoxybenzamine is an α-adrenoceptor blocker which is effective at treating these symptoms of sympathetic overactivity. Surgical resection of the tumour is needed for definitive treatment.

Dental aspects
Phaeochromocytoma is occasionally associated with oral mucosal neuromas (multiple endocrine adenoma (MEA) type III syndrome). Patients who have had adrenal surgery for phaeochromocytoma may suffer from hypoadrenocorticism, since the adrenal cortex is inevitably damaged at operation. These patients therefore require steroid cover at operation.

Five facts

1. The adrenal cortex secretes steroid hormones (such as glucocorticoids, mineralocorticoids and sex steroids).
2. The adrenal medulla secretes catecholamines (such as adrenaline, noradrenaline and dopamine).
3. Patients on long-term steroid treatment need a higher dose during trauma, illness or surgery; otherwise, an adrenal (Addisonian) crisis may occur.
4. An adrenal crisis presents with hypotension, nausea, vomiting, hypoglycaemia and drowsiness/coma.
5. Patients on long-term steroids receiving dental treatment have prolonged wound healing and increased risk of infection.

Allergy and anaphylaxis

Allergy is the intolerance of the body to a specific substance due to an immune response to a specific antigen. An allergy can range in severity from a nuisance to a life-threatening emergency (anaphylaxis). Common allergies include asthma, hayfever and eczema. Allergies to drugs or foods such as peanuts may occur and can be life-threatening. Certain individuals and families are *atopic*. Atopic individuals are at higher risk of developing certain allergies such as asthma, hayfever and eczema.

Pathology

Allergic reactions may be classified into two main types of immune response.

Type I (immediate) hypersensitivity
Hayfever, asthma and eczema are examples of type I hypersensitivity. Allergies to pollen, dust mites, mould and pet dander are common causes of hayfever (allergic rhinitis) and asthma. Other common allergens are milk and egg proteins, but in many cases the allergen cannot be reliably identified. Such allergic reactions are related to antibodies of the immunoglobulin E (IgE) class. The first time an allergy-prone individual is exposed to an allergen, the individual makes large amounts of the corresponding IgE antibody. This attaches to basophils (in the circulation) and to mast cells, which are plentiful in the lungs, skin, tongue and linings of the nose and intestinal tract. When exposure of a sensitized individual to an antigen occurs, it binds to the antibodies, and triggers almost immediate mast cell degranulation with histamine release. This causes, within minutes, itching, vasodilatation, increased capillary permeability and swelling and may also cause bronchoconstriction.

Type IV (delayed) hypersensitivity
Contact dermatitis is an example of a type IV hypersensitivity reaction. Many cases of latex allergy are of this type. When exposure of a sensitized individual to an antigen occurs, a response mediated by T lymphocytes is triggered, causing inflammation. This response may take several hours.

Clinical features

Allergic rhinitis (hayfever)
Allergic rhinitis is a type IV hypersensitivity reaction to pollen from various plants that is characterized by mucoid nasal discharge, an itchy nose and sneezing. Associated conjunctivitis produces itchy, runny eyes.

Eczema
Eczema is an allergic reaction of the skin. Localized itching and irritation of the skin is characteristic. Eczema manifests acutely with swelling, redness with papules and vesicles. Chronically, the skin may thicken (lichenification). Atopic eczema is a type I hypersensitivity to allergens such as pollen and house dust mite. Contact

eczema/dermatitis is a type IV hypersensitivity reaction produced by direct and prolonged contact (several hours) with various substances such as nickel or perfume.

Anaphylaxis
Anaphylaxis is an acute, severe and systemic type I hypersensitivity reaction which may be life-threatening. Clinically, skin manifestations include erythema and urticaria (acute swelling in the skin). Conjunctivitis and rhinitis may also occur. Bronchospasm and laryngeal obstruction may occur and cause acute obstruction of upper and lower airways, respectively. Hypotension, tachycardia and shock also develop.

Asthma
See chapter on asthma.

Investigations

Patch tests
Patch tests are used to test allergens for a type IV hypersensitivity reaction. Discs impregnated with one allergen each are held against the skin for 24–48 hours. Any eczematous reaction seen afterwards indicates an allergy.

Skin prick tests
About 10–20 common allergens (antigens which mediate allergy via type I hypersensitivity) are tested. Using needles, allergens are individually impregnated into the skin of the forearm, at certain points. After 20 min, any allergens to which the individual is sensitive will show an eczematous reaction.

RAST
The radioallergosorbent test (RAST) is an alternative to skin prick testing. A range of specific IgEs to various allergens may be assayed in the serum of an individual. If the level of the RAST to one specific allergen is raised, then that individual has an allergy to it.

Management of allergy

Allergen avoidance
Allergen avoidance is vital to successful treatment. Allergies, e.g. to pets or food, may therefore be controlled effectively but not all allergens, e.g. pollen, can be avoided effectively.

Antihistamines
Systemic or topical (e.g. skin, eye or nose) H_1 antagonists (e.g. chlorphenamine) are useful in antagonizing the effects of type I hypersensitivity reactions. The major side effect is drowsiness. Loratidine and desloratidine are less sedating.

Corticosteroids
Systemic or topical steroids are useful in treating all types of allergic reaction.

Management of anaphylaxis

Anaphylaxis is a medical emergency:

1. Always call for urgent medical attention without delay.
2. Airway: laryngeal obstruction produces stridor. If it occurs, emergency intubation should be performed by an anaesthetist. If this is not available, a cricothyroidotomy should be performed immediately, and a 14G cannula inserted into it in order to produce an airway.
3. High-flow oxygen.
4. Intramuscular (IM) adrenaline (epinephrine) 0.5–1 ml (1 in 1000 strength) should be administered without delay.
5. Intravenous (IV) chlorphenamine 10–20 mg.
6. IV hydrocortisone 200 mg.
7. If the patient is hypotensive, IV fluids should be given.

Dental aspects

- Allergic reactions may arise to materials or drugs used in dentistry. The patient and/or dental staff can be affected. If there is a history of allergy to a drug or material, it must be avoided.
- Allergic reactions to latex and rubber products have become increasingly common since the widespread use of protective medical gloves following the advent of AIDS. Latex allergies are common in patients frequently exposed to medical gloves during care, or chronically exposed to latex because of urethral catheterization. Non-patient groups who appear to be at higher risk of sensitization include anyone with dermatitis, since this can facilitate the transfer of antigens across the skin. Allergy to latex is now the main allergic occupational problem for health care workers.
- Latex exposure can be via the skin, mucous membranes, or respiratory system via inhaled latex glove powder. Some of the allergens may also be associated with the glove lubricating powder, and may become aerosolized, causing respiratory, ocular or nasal symptoms. Latex is found in many items used in clinics, wards and operating theatres apart from gloves, including:
  - rubber dam
  - intubation tubes
  - anaesthetic masks and other anaesthetic equipment
  - catheters
  - tourniquets
  - sphygmomanometer cuffs
  - rubber surgical drains
  - stethoscopes.
- Hypersensitivity reactions to beta-lactam antibiotics (penicillins and cephalosporins) are the most frequent type of immunological reactions to drugs and are more likely to follow perenteral rather than oral administration. Patients allergic to penicillin can usually react to any other penicillin except aztreonam, and sometimes also react to cephalosporins. A history of previous reactions to penicillin suggests a greater risk of acute anaphylaxis but there is no completely

reliable method of prediction.
- Aspirin can provoke allergic reactions, albeit rarely. Aspirin-induced asthma is a recognized but rare side effect, mainly in patients with nasal polyps ('triad asthma' – asthma, nasal polyps and aspirin sensitivity).
- Allergic reactions to local anaesthetic agents such as lidocaine (lignocaine) are highly questionable.

Five facts

1. Allergy is an immune response to a specific antigen (an allergen).
2. Asthma, eczema and hayfever are all types of allergy.
3. Allergen avoidance is the best management of allergy.
4. Anaphylaxis is an acute, severe, systemic allergy which may produce hypotension, bronchospasm, laryngeal obstruction, skin urticaria and erythema.
5. Acute management of anaphylaxis includes protection of the airway, IM adrenaline (epinephrine), IV hydrocortisone and IV chlorphenamine (antihistamine).

Anaemia

The carriage of oxygen from the lungs to the rest of the body, and carbon dioxide back to the lungs is essential for life. Oxygen is carried in the blood by haemoglobin (Hb), which is found in red blood cells in the blood. A single molecule of adult haemoglobin (HbA) in the adult consists of four polypeptide chains (two alpha chains and two beta chains), each with its own haem molecule. A molecule of haem is made from the combination of protoporphyrin to an atom of iron.

Red blood cells (RBCs) or erythrocytes are produced in the bone marrow. Numerous substances are necessary for the biosynthesis of erythrocytes, including metals (iron, cobalt, manganese), vitamins (B_{12}, B_6, C, E, folate, riboflavin, pantothenic acid, thiamine) and amino acids. Regulatory substances necessary for normal erythropoiesis include erythropoietin, thyroid hormones and androgens.

Anaemia is an abnormally low level of haemoglobin in the blood; this for an adult is less than 12–13 g/dl. Anaemia is extremely common. Women are more affected than men, due to physiological blood loss during menstruation. **Anaemia is not in itself a diagnosis, and should always be investigated for its underlying cause.**

Classification of anaemia

Anaemia is classified according to the RBC size: mean cell volume (MCV) = haematocrit/RBC count. The haematocrit (packed cell volume or PCV) is a measure of the total volume of the RBC relative to the total volume of whole blood in a sample.

Anaemia is therefore classified into:

- microcytic anaemia – MCV <85 fl
- normocytic anaemia – MCV 85–98 fl
- macrocytic anaemia – MCV >98 fl.

Clinical features of anaemia

Most individuals with anaemia are completely asymptomatic, since they can tolerate a lower than normal level of haemoglobin. However, at lower levels of haemoglobin and in individuals with coexisting disease, symptoms may occur, including fatigue and shortness of breath on exertion. These may manifest as decreased exercise tolerance, e.g. on climbing stairs. Exertional angina and cardiac failure may arise in individuals with pre-existing heart disease. General signs of anaemia are pallor of the conjunctivae and skin. Tachycardia, tachypnoea and signs of heart failure may be present.

Microcytic (hypochromic) anaemias

Iron deficiency anaemia
Iron (Fe) deficiency is the most common cause of anaemia. It may produce koilonychia (spooning of the nails) and angular stomatitis (inflammation at the angle of the mouth). Iron deficiency anaemia is most commonly caused by chronic blood loss. However, it may also be caused by inadequate dietary intake or by malabsorption.

Chronic blood loss
The most common site of blood loss is the gastrointestinal (GI) tract, from lesions such as a peptic ulcer, a neoplasm, e.g. colon cancer, or angiodysplasia (abnormal blood vessels in the colon with a tendency to bleed). Therefore, a history of haematemesis (vomiting blood), rectal bleeding, or melaena (black, tar-like faeces) should be sought. Weight loss, change in bowel habit and tenesmus (sensation of incomplete emptying of bowels) may suggest colon cancer. A rectal examination is mandatory and colonoscopy may then be indicated.

Other sites of chronic blood loss are the urine, or the uterus during menstruation. It is common for women of reproductive age to be mildly iron deficient due to menstruation.

Malabsorption
Iron is absorbed in the small intestine, and therefore coeliac disease may cause iron deficiency.

Treatment
Iron deficiency is treated with oral iron supplementation.

Thalassaemia
Thalassaemias are genetic diseases characterized by low production of either the alpha or beta chain of Hb. Most cases of *beta-thalassaemia* are seen in individuals of Mediterranean, Indian and Arabic origin. *Beta-thalassaemia major* is a serious homozygous defect, leading to almost no beta chains; HbA is vastly reduced, with severe anaemia. *Beta-thalassaemia minor* is due to a heterozygous defect causing only mild anaemia. *Alpha-thalassaemia* is mainly found in the Far East, Middle East and Africa. Mutations in all four alpha chain genes lead to stillbirth (*hydrops fetalis*), three mutations cause an intermediate severity of *alpha-thalassaemia* and two mutations cause *alpha-thalassaemia minor*.

Complications of thalassaemias include marrow hyperplasia, splenomegaly and iron overload from repeated blood transfusions. Treatment of thalassaemia major consists of regular blood transfusions given with desferrioxamine to prevent iron overload and secondary haemochromatosis. Splenectomy may be performed in severe cases to reduce the need for blood transfusion.

Sideroblastic anaemia
Sideroblastic anaemia is a condition caused by defects in haem synthesis. It leads to iron overload and therefore the formation in the bone marrow of ring sideroblasts (erythrocytes with a ring of iron-containing granules). Sideroblastic anaemia may be due to a hereditary defect in haem synthesis or it may be acquired (myelodysplasia or drugs, e.g. isoniazid).

Lead poisoning
Lead interferes with haem synthesis and therefore reduces the production of haemoglobin. Lead causes the precipitation of denatured RNA in the erythrocyte cytoplasm, leading to basophilic stippling seen on examination of the blood film.

Normocytic (normochromic) anaemias

Anaemia of chronic disease

Decreased utilization of iron stores or decreased erythropoiesis in any chronic disease may cause anaemia.

Sickle cell anaemia (SCA)

Sickle cell anaemia is predominantly seen in people of Afro-Caribbean origin but may be seen in Arabs, Greeks, Italians, Latin Americans, and individuals from India. SCA is an inherited Hb defect (haemoglobinopathy) due to a defect in the structure of the beta chain. Hb electrophoresis is needed to detect the sickled Hb (HbS); this tells if the patient has the *disease* or is a carrier of the sickle cell *trait* (see below). HbS polymerizes at low oxygen tensions, resulting in sickle-shaped RBCs.

Sickle cells block capillaries, and therefore may lead to several clinical 'crises':

- Vaso-occlusive crisis – due to bone ischaemia, e.g. femur, hands (dactylitis).
- Splenic (sequestration) crisis – occlusion of venous drainage from the spleen causes painful splenomegaly which is susceptible to rupture and sequesters RBCs. The spleen eventually infarcts (autosplenectomy), making individuals susceptible to infection from capsulated bacteria such as pneumococcus, meningococcus and haemophilus. Vaccination and lifelong prophylactic penicillin V are used to prevent infection.
- Sickle chest crisis – pulmonary infarction and respiratory failure occur due to sickle cells trapped in the lung vasculature.
- Oxygen, rehydration and opioids may be required for the above.
- Aplastic crisis – bone marrow aplasia precipitated by parvovirus B19 infection.

Complications of sickle cell anaemia can thus include:

- pain episodes
- strokes
- increased infections
- leg ulcers
- bone damage
- yellow eyes or jaundice
- early gallstones
- lung damage
- kidney damage
- painful sustained erections in men (priapism)
- blood blockage in the spleen or liver (sequestration)
- eye damage
- anaemia
- delayed growth.

Sickle cell *trait* is seen in heterozygotes; it is more common than SCA, but less severe. It may cause significant illness during times of stress such as surgery. Interestingly, sickle cell trait confers a degree of protection from malaria.

Haemolysis

Inherited haemolytic anaemias:
- Hereditary spherocytosis – caused by mutations in RBC membrane proteins (e.g. ankyrin). Abnormally spherical RBCs have a reduced life span. Hereditary elliptocytosis is a less severe version of the same condition.
- Glucose-6-phosphate dehydrogenase (G6PD) deficiency causes increased susceptibility of RBCs to drug-induced oxidative damage, e.g. by dapsone and sulphonamides.
- Pyruvate kinase deficiency reduces ATP production, causing haemolysis.

Acquired haemolytic anaemias
Autoimmune haemolytic anaemia is caused by autoantibody-mediated RBC destruction:

- warm autoimmune haemolytic anaemia, associated with infectious mononucleosis, SLE (systemic lupus erythematosus) and lymphoma, is caused by IgM (immunoglobulin M), which is most active at 37°C.
- cold autoimmune haemolytic anaemia, associated with *Mycoplasma* and lymphoma, is mediated by IgG, which is most active at 4°C.

Autoimmune haemolytic anaemia should improve with treatment of the underlying disease. Oral prednisolone is usually given. Splenectomy may be needed in unresponsive cases.

Other acquired haemolytic anaemias
Mechanical heart valves may cause haemolysis via turbulence of blood. Microangiopathic haemolytic anaemia is associated with haemolytic uraemic syndrome (HUS) and thrombotic thrombocytopenic purpura (TTP). It causes fibrin deposition in capillaries, which directly leads to RBC destruction.

Macrocytic (hyperchromic) anaemias

Vitamin B$_{12}$ deficiency
Vitamin B$_{12}$ and folate are essential for the conversion of homocysteine into methionine, which is needed for the synthesis of DNA. Vitamin B$_{12}$ and folate deficiency may therefore produce anaemia, as well as thrombocytopenia and leukopenia. Vitamin B$_{12}$ deficiency anaemia may produce glossitis and can lead to peripheral neuropathy, including subacute combined degeneration of the spinal cord.

Vitamin B$_{12}$ binds to intrinsic factor (IF), which is secreted by parietal cells in the stomach. Pancreatic enzymes are required for binding of vitamin B$_{12}$ to IF. Vitamin B$_{12}$ is then absorbed in the terminal ileum bound to IF. Vitamin B$_{12}$ malabsorption may therefore be caused by gastric pathology (e.g. pernicious anaemia, partial gastrectomy or gastritis), pancreatic insufficiency or terminal ileal disease (e.g. Crohn's disease). Dietary deficiency of vitamin B$_{12}$ is uncommon since it takes 3 years for liver stores to become depleted.

Treatment is with 3-monthly hydroxocobalamin (vitamin B$_{12}$) injections.

Folate deficiency

Folate deficiency anaemia may produce glossitis. States of high red cell turnover, such as puberty and pregnancy, may lead to folate deficiency. Dietary folate deficiency is caused by poor vegetable intake. Since folate is absorbed in the small intestine, coeliac disease may also cause its deficiency. Drugs such as azathioprine and methotrexate inhibit folate metabolism, thereby limiting DNA synthesis.

Treatment is with oral folate.

Investigations of anaemia

Full blood count

Full blood count gives a measurement of the level of Hb, and the MCV.

Blood film

Blood film may give valuable information as to the cause of anaemia. Iron deficiency anaemia may produce anisocytosis (different sizes of RBCs), poikilocytosis (different shapes of RBCs), pencil cells and target cells. Vitamin B_{12}/folate deficiency may show neutrophil hypersegmentation on blood film examination. Sickle cells may be seen in sickle cell anaemia.

Iron studies

A low ferritin, low serum Fe, high TIBC (total iron binding capacity) and low transferrin saturation index indicates iron deficiency.

Vitamin B_{12}/folate

Low serum vitamin B_{12} levels are diagnostic of vitamin B_{12} deficiency. Since serum folate levels are highly variable, RBC folate levels are a better measure.

Haemoglobin electrophoresis

Haemoglobin electrophoresis is used to detect mutations of thalassaemia and sickle cell anaemia.

Direct Coombs' (antiglobulin) test

This test is performed to diagnose autoimmune haemolytic anaemia. The patient's RBCs (which are coated in autoantibodies in autoimmune haemolytic anaemia) are mixed with the Coombs' reagent which contains antibodies to human IgG and IgM. Coombs' antibodies will bind to the autoantibodies on the RBCs, therefore causing RBC agglutination only in autoimmune haemolytic anaemia.

Upper and lower gastrointestinal endoscopy

Upper and lower GI endoscopy is important in the investigation of iron deficiency anaemia in order to detect blood loss.

Bone marrow examination

If any dysplasia is present in blood cells, then the bone marrow should be examined for evidence of myelodysplasia or leukaemia. Bone marrow iron stores can also be assessed.

Management of anaemia

Treatment should be aimed at the underlying cause. For example, in iron deficiency this would be identifying any site of possible latent bleeding. However, if symptoms are severe (e.g. shortness of breath on minimal exertion, angina), then a blood transfusion should be given. Folate supplementation should also be given for any anaemia with a high turnover of cells (e.g. haemolytic anaemia).

Genetic screening/counselling

If both parents are carriers for an inherited anaemia, e.g. sickle cell, genetic analysis of fetal tissue using chorionic villous sampling may be performed to see if the fetus is homozygous. However, the decision to perform this procedure and possibly terminate the fetus must be made by the parents.

Dental aspects

Some anaemias can cause oral complaints:

- ulcers, burning mouth syndrome, glossitis or angular stomatitis in deficiency anaemias
- jaw expansion from bone marrow hyperplasia in haemolytic anaemias
- pain from infarcts in sickle cell anaemia.

Whenever possible, anaemia should be corrected preoperatively if general anaesthesia is to be used – if necessary, by transfusion.

Five facts

1. Anaemia is an abnormally low level of haemoglobin in the blood (typically below 12–13 g/dl).
2. Anaemia is classified according to the size of red blood cells (microcytic, normocytic or macrocytic).
3. Clinical features of anaemia include fatigue, shortness of breath on exertion, exertional angina, pale skin and pale conjunctivae.
4. Anaemia is *not* in itself a diagnosis, and the underlying cause must always be investigated.
5. The most common cause of anaemia is iron deficiency anaemia (mostly due to menstrual or gastrointestinal bleeding).

Anaesthesia and sedation

Local anaesthetics

Local anaesthetic (LA) molecules bind specifically to sodium channel proteins in axonal membranes of neurons near the injection site, with essentially no effects centrally unless given in overdose. Local anaesthetics are all weak bases, and exist *in vivo* in both their ionized and unionized forms. The degree of ionization depends on the pH of the solution they exist in and on their own pKa (the pH at which the ionized and unionized forms exist in equal concentrations). They act by blocking the sodium channels that generate action potentials. The local anaesthetic molecule which is deposited outside the nerve fibre must cross the lipid axon membrane to exert its effect. Hence, the molecule must exist in its unionized form and be lipid soluble. The more lipid soluble the drug, the more potent it will be. Also, as different local anaesthetics have different pKa values, they will consequently have different speeds of onset of action.

The first LA was discovered over 100 years ago and the early ones included cocaine, procaine and derivatives known as ester-type LAs. Commonly used agents nowadays include the amides – lignocaine (recently renamed lidocaine), articaine mepivicaine, bupivacaine and prilocaine. All share a common chemical structure, with an amide group joined to an aromatic group by a linking group.

Dentists are permitted to use LA, but should be careful to never exceed safe dose limits. The most commonly used agent is lidocaine (rapid onset of action, moderate potency), which has a safe dose limit of 3 mg/kg (i.e. 10.5 ml 2% for a 70 kg man). The addition of adrenaline (epinephrine) to local anaesthetics allows a greater amount of LA to be given (7 mg/kg for lidocaine) and is used for its vasoconstrictory properties to minimize bleeding. However, this same vasoconstriction can lead to gangrene and necrosis if used on end arteries, and thus adrenaline should never be used on the extremities like fingers or the penis (except by careful anaesthetists!). Felypressin is a synthetic analogue of vasopressin sometimes used with prilocaine, with little of the antidiuretic or oxytocin-like actions of vasopressin. Even if given intravenously in amounts far in excess of those used for local anaesthesia, felypressin has little toxicity. The administration of large amounts of felypressin to patients receiving general anaesthesia with halothane may result in cyanosis and a slight rise in blood pressure, but these changes are not serious.

Whenever LA is used, at whatever dose, there should be great care not to inject intravenously, and the patient should be observed for signs of toxicity, typically affecting the brain and heart. Cerebral toxicity most seriously manifests as convulsions, although there is usually preceding confusion and excitement. Cardiovascular effects include bradycardia and arrhythmias. Bupivacaine is notorious for its cardiac toxicity and thus it is gradually being replaced with its safer optical isomer, ropivacaine.

Conscious sedation

Nitrous oxide plus oxygen is overall the safest combination for conscious sedation because of its lack of respiratory or cardiodepressant effects, and rapid reversibility.

The benzodiazepines are also useful for conscious sedation. They are mild respiratory depressants with minimal risk to healthy persons, although potentially dangerous to those with cardiorespiratory disease and particularly chronic obstructive pulmonary disease. Midazolam is considerably (2 or 3 times) more potent than diazepam and the onset of signs of sedation is less reliable. The maximal effect of midazolam on the brain appears to be about 10–15 min after intravenous administration. As a consequence, there have been a few deaths after administration of midazolam alone in elderly patients. Cases have been reported of potentiation of midazolam by erythromycin. Flumazenil may be used to reverse the effect of midazolam.

Propofol appears to have the advantages of a rapid sedative response, with a quicker recovery and better effects on mood compared with midazolam.

Fantasies of sexual assault may arise during benzodiazepine sedation, and thus it is essential that sedation is not administered in the absence of a second trained person.

General anaesthesia

General anaesthesia (GA) is a triad of:

- anaesthesia (making the patient unconscious)
- analgesia (pain relief)
- muscle relaxation (to facilitate surgery that would be impeded by muscle tone).

All of the above three elements are necessary for the surgeon to operate successfully. The advent of GA has led to major advances in surgical practice that would otherwise have been impossible. In fact, it was a dentist who was the first to administer general anaesthesia in the form of ether.

Nowadays, an anaesthetist should administer a GA; indeed no untrained physician, dentist or surgeon should. Non-adherence to this rule has led to many unnecessary deaths. GA for dental purposes must now be given only in hospital.

There are many GA preparations in current practice, and they can be broadly classified according to their route of administration. Gaseous preparations such as halothane are widely used, but intravenous thiopental or propofol are usually the gold standard.

Before GA, the patient must take no food for 6 hours, but clear fluids can be taken up to 3 hours (adult) or 2 hours (child) before operation. This is to avoid the possible vomiting and inhalation of vomit that can arise in GA.

Muscle relaxation can be achieved by the use of depolarizing agents (such as suxamethonium) or non-depolarizing agents (such as atracurium or vecuronium). The distinction is based on the fact that suxamethonium activates the nicotinic acetylcholine (ACh) receptor, mimicking the action of ACh, whereas the non-depolarizing drugs are all competitive inhibitors of ACh at the nicotinic ACh receptor and do not stimulate it. Suxamethonium has a quicker onset of action but its effect does not last as long as the non-depolarizing neuromuscular blockers. Also, the side effects of suxamethonium are many, whereas the non-depolarizers achieve pure skeletal muscle paralysis. A few patients lack the enzyme necessary to break down suxamethonium and then suffer apnoea if given the drug (scoline sensitivity).

Muscle relaxants are also used by anaesthetists for purposes other than facilitating surgery. For example, they can help facilitate endotracheal intubation in sedated patients and limit muscle contractions during the convulsions induced by electroconvulsive therapy. As with other anaesthetic agents these drugs should only be administered by a trained anaesthetist.

The analgesics used when patients are given general anaesthesia are also a matter for the anaesthetist, but opiate use is common.

Dental aspects

- Dentists can provide local anaesthesia and conscious sedation.
- If working in hospital, dentists may be required to assess patients for GA, to ensure essential prerequisites are met before GA. They may need to manage postoperative care and therefore they must have an understanding of perioperative care.
- LA is remarkably safe if given in safe doses with an aspirating syringe. Drug interactions with LA are rare. Allergy to LA agents is exceedingly rare, but sulphites or other preservatives may be sensitizing. Tens of thousands of dental LA are given daily with no untoward effects.
- In conducting conscious sedation in the UK, the requirements of the Code of Practice issued by the General Dental Council must be fulfilled. There is no place for the operator-anaesthetist, and conscious sedation should only be carried out with well-trained staff and suitable equipment for life support. All patients must be monitored perioperatively, clinically and with a pulse oximeter and blood pressure monitor.

Precautions before conscious sedation or general anaesthesia

Patients quickly forget or fail to take in what they are told. Therefore, it is important not merely to give instructions verbally, but also to give these same instructions in written form when it has been decided that either general anaesthesia or sedation is necessary.

Identification of the patient and operation site

The patient's name and the reason for having general anaesthesia must be confirmed. This apparently obvious precaution avoids embarrassing confusion between patients coming from a crowded waiting room. The operation site should be marked in ink, by the operator, while the patient is conscious, and checked with the patient.

Informed consent

Written consent to general anaesthesia must be obtained before each operation. Suitable consent forms are supplied by the medical defence societies. It is also helpful, and there is increasing pressure, to provide patients with written information relevant to their treatment.

No food or drink

Adults should not consume food or take oral medication for 6 hours preoperatively. Food or materials present in the stomach may be vomited and inhaled during anaesthesia, with disastrous consequences. Clear instructions must be given that adults should take no food or drink (including tea or alcohol) for 6 hours preoperatively, although clear fluids may be taken up to 3 hours preoperatively. Clear fluids include still water or fruit squash, not tea, coffee, milk, fizzy drinks or alcohol. Vomiting is more likely in a patient who is pregnant or has gastric disease or a head injury, or has taken alcohol or a drug such as erythromycin which may precipitate vomiting.

In the case of children, however, it is important to avoid dehydration, and thus clear fluids can be taken up to 2 hours before the anaesthetic. However, food should not be taken for 6 hours preoperatively.

Dentures, bladder, bowels and other factors

Dentures should be removed preoperatively. The anaesthetist must be warned of the presence of crowned, fragile or loose teeth, or bridges which could be damaged during intubation, of contact lenses, hearing aids, or a colostomy bag. The bladder should be emptied preoperatively and it is sometimes necessary to catheterize inpatients. A nasogastric tube should be inserted if required. It may be necessary to shave a skin operation site. Never shave eyebrows.

Psychological preparation and premedication

Most people are apprehensive of general anaesthesia; some are terrified. Dental treatment in general, and oral surgery in particular, is stressful for many patients, and can induce a rise in blood pressure and pulse rate, as well as ECG changes. Apart from poor cooperation as a result of anxiety, autonomic overactivity can precipitate cardiac arrhythmias, swings in blood pressure and vomiting.

One of the most effective methods of reducing anxiety is by sympathetic reassurance and brief discussion of a patient's particular anxieties. If this fails, however, premedication with a benzodiazepine may be necessary, although this is not usually feasible in general dental practice as it delays recovery. Benzodiazepines may also be ineffective in children and in patients on long-term medication with psychoactive drugs.

Anaesthetists vary widely in their requirements for premedication. The main purpose of premedication is to lessen anxiety, and it is typically given 30–35 min preoperatively. For inpatients, benzodiazepines or opioids (pethidine, morphine or Omnopon), are traditional premedicants because of their sedative action. However, opioids increase nausea, vomiting and respiratory depression. Promethazine or alimemazine may be used for their sedative and antiemetic effect, and for premedication of children, but they have a prolonged action and are often ineffective. They also raise blood sugar levels – a consideration when treating diabetics. Children may be given oral alimemazine or triclofos, or rectal barbiturates such as thiopental.

Benzodiazepines are useful because of their anxiolytic and amnesic actions. The relative freedom from side effects and the wide safety margin have caused diazepam, lorazepam and temazepam to become increasingly widely used. Beta-blockers may also be used and may help to prevent dysrhythmias induced by surgery.

Atropinics such as atropine, glycopyrronium or hyoscine are antiemetics and may also reduce the parasympathomimetic effects and dysrhythmias sometimes associated with suxamethonium but are unlikely to be needed for outpatients. However, the effectiveness of atropinics in preventing dysrhythmias other than vagal overactivity is controversial. Glaucoma is a specific contraindication to the use of atropinics and diazepam. Since the maximal effect of atropine is apparent 30–60 min after injection, some anaesthetists give the drug during induction of anaesthesia, thus achieving the desired parasympatholytic effect during the operation while sparing the patient the unpleasant dry mouth and thirst during the preoperative period. Hyoscine is best avoided in the elderly in whom it may cause confusion. Atropinics should not be given to febrile patients.

Benzodiazepines give sedation with amnesia but no analgesia. Give slowly intravenously and then give local analgesia. Diazepam may cause pain or thrombophlebitis, and drowsiness returns transiently 4–6 hours postoperatively due to metabolism to oxazepam and desmethyldiazepam and enterohepatic recirculation. It may produce mild hypotension and respiratory depression. Midazolam, compared to diazepam, has a quicker onset of action, and amnesia is more profound, with more rapid recovery, and lower incidence of venous thrombosis.

After conscious sedation or GA, the immediate postoperative period is the most dangerous. Great care of the airway must be ensured. A responsible adult must accompany the recovered patient home. The patient must not drive or ride any vehicle, operate unguarded machinery, or make important decisions until 24 hours after any operation under conscious sedation or GA. Deaths as a result of the use of general anaesthesia in the dental surgery have been few, but nevertheless have provoked widespread public concern. As a result of legislation, it is no longer feasible in the UK for the dentist to act as anaesthetist, and this has been the case for some time in certain other countries. GA must only be given in a hospital with critical care facilities because of the need to have resuscitatory equipment available.

Five facts

1. The maximum safe dose of lidocaine (lignocaine) is 3 mg/kg (21 ml 1% for a 70 kg man).
2. Adrenaline (epinephrine) should not be used on the extremities without extreme caution.
3. GA is a triad of anaesthesia, analgesia and muscle relaxation.
4. GA for dental purposes must only be given in hospital.
5. After conscious sedation or GA, care of the airway is essential and a responsible adult should accompany the patient home.

Arthritis

Arthritis is a term for joint disorders that cause *pain*, *deformity* and *limitation of movement*.

Osteoarthritis

Osteoarthritis (OA) is the most common form of arthritis. OA is a non-inflammatory/degenerative symmetrical polyarthropathy which most commonly affects *large* joints such as the hips, knees and shoulders. It can also affect the hands, especially the distal interphalangeal (DIP) joints. Bony lumps may appear on the fingers, on the proximal interphalangeal (PIP) joints (Bouchard's nodes) or DIP joints (Heberden's nodes), or the 1st metacarpophalangeal (MCP) joint at the thumb base. There are no extra-articular features.

There is a strong female predominance and most cases affect older individuals. Most cases of OA are idiopathic, but some cases have an identified cause which leads to increased joint wear – such as obesity, trauma (e.g. footballer injuries) or occupation (e.g. athletics).

The pathology of OA involves chondrocyte activation, which leads to thinning of the cartilage layer over the joint and narrowing of the joint space. The underlying bone develops cysts and osteophytes (bony outgrowths into the joint).

Rheumatoid arthritis

Rheumatoid arthritis (RA) is the commonest form of inflammatory arthropathy. RA is much more common in women and the onset is typically in adulthood, between 20 and 40 years old. RA is mainly a symmetrical *small* joint arthropathy. The MCP joints, wrists, elbows and ankles are most commonly affected. The DIP joints are characteristically spared. Ulnar deviation at the MCP joints is caused by subluxation of the joints. Synovial effusions and rheumatoid nodules may also be found. Extra-articular features may include eye involvement (mainly conjunctivitis), lung lesions (pleural effusion, pleural plaques), pericarditis and Sjögren's syndrome.

RA is an autoimmune disorder associated with various autoantibodies (i.e. it is often 'seropositive'). This means the presence of rheumatoid factor (IgM to the Fc portion of IgG), when the disease is more aggressive. A destructive synovitis develops with infiltration predominantly by CD4 T lymphocytes. Genetic factors are important, and there is genetic linkage to the alleles HLA-DR4 and HLA-DR-1.

Seronegative spondyloarthropathies

This is a group of arthritides in which autoantibodies are not found, and which are united by certain clinical features, which include:

- Asymmetrical arthritis, particularly affecting axial joints.
- Enthesopathy: inflammation of the junction between tendon and bone.

- Extra-articular features:
  - eye – conjunctivitis, anterior uveitis
  - heart – cardiac arrhythmias, aortic incompetence
  - skin – pustular lesions.

These arthritides are characterized by extrasynovial inflammation of joints. There is a strong association with HLA-B27. However, most people with HLA-B27 do *not* have a seronegative spondyloarthropathy, which means that the detection of HLA-B27 is of no practical diagnostic value.

Specific seronegative spondyloarthropathies are described in Table 1.

Table 1 Specific seronegative spondyloarthropathies, together with main associations and features

Arthropathy	Associations	Main features
Ankylosing spondylitis	>90% HLA-B27	Sacroiliitis, spondylosis (fusion of spinal vertebrae)
Reactive arthritis (formerly termed Reiter's syndrome)	Non-gonococcal urethritis or colitis, e.g. salmonella, shigella, yersinia	Triad of: 1. conjunctivitis 2. arthritis 3. urethritis
Psoriatic arthritis	Psoriasis	Skin: salmon pink plaques Nails: thimble pitting, onycholysis (thickening of the nail)
Enteropathy-associated arthritis	Inflammatory bowel disease (IBD)	Predominantly lower limb arthritis, which improves with treatment of IBD

Crystal arthropathies

The two main arthropathies caused by deposition of crystals in joints are gout and pseudogout.

Gout

Gout has a strong predominance in men and is caused by hyperuricaemia, which results from an imbalance between urate production (from the breakdown of purine nucleotides)/ingestion and urate excretion. Urate crystals are deposited in the joints (*negatively* birefringent under polarized light).

Gout most commonly affects the first metatarsophalangeal (MTP) joint, but can affect other small joints such as the ankle, wrist, knee and small joints of the hand. In acute gout, a single joint is affected and may be difficult to distinguish from septic arthritis, which is a surgical emergency. There is a rapid onset of extreme pain, swelling, erythema and hotness of the joint, which may last for 1–2 weeks.

Chronic tophaceous gout produces chronic pain and is characterized by the presence of gouty tophi (subcutaneous deposits of urate crystals) in the fingers, elbows or the cartilage of the ears.

Pseudogout
Pseudogout is caused by deposition of calcium pyrophosphate (*positively* birefringent under polarized light). The acute clinical features are indistinguishable from gout. Associations include osteoarthritis, hyperparathyroidism, hypophosphataemia and haemochromatosis.

Septic arthritis

Infection is the most serious cause of arthritis, since, without treatment, there can be rapid, irreversible joint damage. Septic arthritis may be clinically indistinguishable from other acute arthritides such as acute gout. The affected joint is hot, swollen and painful, and the overlying skin is erythematous. Bacterial infection may spread to the joint by direct inoculation (e.g. trauma or surgical procedure) or via the blood (haematological spread). Commonly involved bacteria include *Staphylococcus aureus* (from skin trauma or direct spread), gonococcus (urethritis) or streptococcus (wounds, respiratory tract).

If septic arthritis is suspected, the joint should be drained *immediately* under aseptic conditions followed by microscopy for organisms and empirical intravenous (IV) antibiotics.

Investigations in arthritis

Plain X-rays of the joints
Anterior-posterior and lateral views of the joints should be performed in order to aid diagnosis of the type of arthritis, as well as the extent of disease involvement.

Serum inflammatory markers
Serum inflammatory markers such as C-reactive protein (CRP) and erythrocyte sedimentation rate (ESR) are non-specific markers of inflammation which may be used to monitor disease activity, and to measure response to treatment.

Serum immunology
Rheumatoid factor (RF) (as discussed above).

Serum biochemical markers
Serum urate is often raised in gout. Deranged bone metabolism (e.g. raised calcium, low phosphate) may be present in pseudogout.

Joint aspiration
Joint aspiration is a simple and valuable investigation. Microscopy may show organisms with a Gram stain, which diagnoses septic arthritis. Crystals may also be seen under polarized light.

Management in arthritis

Physiotherapy
A programme of regular exercise, together with joint manipulation, is a vital aspect of management. It can help reduce symptoms and maintain the range of movements. Weight control helps minimize stress on joints. A walking stick can ease the load on a damaged hip or knee joint. Heat application may ease pain, relax muscles and increase blood flow to the joint. Cold application may be needed for occasional flare-ups.

Analgesia
Non-steroidal anti-inflammatory drugs (NSAIDs) are the mainstay of pain relief in all types of arthritis.

Control of disease process

Rheumatoid arthritis
DMARDs (disease-modifying antirheumatic drugs) are used to suppress inflammation and prevent disease progression. Methotrexate and sulfasalazine are used as first-line agents. If they are ineffective, other agents should be tried, such as corticosteroids, azathioprine, penicillamine, gold and ciclosporin. These agents are also used to treat severe psoriatic arthropathy.

The side effects of each DMARD are important in determining which one is used for a particular individual.

Gout
Uricosuric drugs
Allopurinol inhibits xanthine oxidase, thus reducing the production of uric acid. It therefore helps to prevent further attacks of gout.

Colchicine
Colchicine acts to inhibit neutrophil microtubule function, and is used in acute gout refractory to NSAID treatment. However, it causes significant side effects of diarrhoea and vomiting.

Septic arthritis
Empirical antibiotic therapy in the absence of any identified source is with IV flucloxacillin (sometimes with IV benzylpenicillin), to cover staphylococci and streptococci.

Surgical treatment
Surgical treatment is used only as a last resort where other measures have failed in controlling joint symptoms or pain from movement. Surgery may be used to replace part or all of a joint (replacement), to fuse a joint (arthrodesis) or to alter the mechanics of a joint (osteotomy). Arthroscopy can be used to remove loose fragments of bone or cartilage that may cause pain or cause mechanical symptoms such as 'locking'.

Dental aspects

- Osteoarthritis affects the temporomandibular joints (TMJ) in some elderly patients but typically painlessly.
- RA may also affect the TMJ, but it is often painless, although there may be stiffness or limitation of opening. Sjögren's syndrome is the main oral complication of RA and causes a dry mouth. In some patients with rheumatoid disease, dislocation of the atlanto-axial joint or fracture of the odontoid peg can readily follow sudden jerking extension of the neck, as a result of weakness of the ligaments.
- Infections of prosthetic joints are usually due to non-oral organisms and only exceptionally rarely to oral bacteria. Antibiotic prophylaxis is therefore not indicated for dental surgery on most patients with bone pins, plates and screws or with total joint replacements but may be considered where dental at-risk procedures (those likely to produce a bacteraemia) are to be carried out in patients who have recent new joints (within 2 years), or in haemophiliacs, or where the joint has previously been infected, or where the patient is immuno-compromised, such as patients with diabetes mellitus.

Five facts

1. Arthritis is defined as inflammation of a joint.
2. If septic arthritis is suspected, IV antibiotics should be started immediately, and an urgent orthopaedic opinion should be sought.
3. Patients with arthritis may be on long-term steroids, which prolong wound healing and predispose the patient to infection and adrenal crisis.
4. Overextension of the neck *must be avoided* in the presence of arthritis, since atlanto-occipital joint dislocation may cause spinal cord compression.
5. Osteoarthritis and rheumatoid arthritis may affect the temporomandibular joints.

Asthma

Asthma and chronic obstructive pulmonary disease (COPD) are the most common lower respiratory disorders. Asthma is a disorder characterized by reversible airways obstruction; it is caused by hyper-reactivity and chronic inflammation of the airways.

Epidemiology

Asthma is common and increasing in prevalence. It affects up to 15% of children and about 5–10% of adults.

Clinical features

Common features are:

- dyspnoea
- wheeze
- chest tightness
- cough.

These symptoms are common to all obstructive airways diseases (such as COPD), but in asthma they are typically variable and episodic in nature. Commonly there is a diurnal pattern, with symptoms and peak expiratory flow rate (PEFR) worst in the mornings. This pattern is referred to as *morning dipping.*

Pathology

Inhalation of allergens (e.g. house dust mite, pollen, smoke) in a sensitized individual results in an inflammatory response that leads to bronchoconstriction. Certain individuals and families are *atopic*, i.e. at higher risk of developing asthma and other allergic diseases (e.g. hayfever, eczema), since they respond to allergens by producing much higher amounts of immunoglobulin E (IgE) than other individuals do.

IgE release produces a type I hypersensitivity reaction, which leads to the production of inflammatory mediators such as histamine and leukotrienes, causing bronchoconstriction. The initial IgE-mediated reaction leads to the recruitment and activation of other cells. These cells, which include T_H2 T lymphocytes via mast cell degranulation, eosinophils, macrophages and epithelial and smooth muscle cells, interact to produce mediators such as interleukins IL-4 and IL-5, which also produce bronchoconstriction. In untreated asthma, in the long term, chronic inflammation occurs, leading to smooth muscle mucous gland hypertrophy and fibrosis of the airways.

Investigations

Peak expiratory flow rate
PEFR is measured using a peak flow meter, which measures the maximum velocity of air expelled by the individual. A lower than normal PEFR is associated with any

type of obstructive airways disease. However, in asthma, the PEFR is *episodically* low.

Spirometry

Spirometry provides measurement of FEV_1 (forced expiratory volume in 1 second) and FVC (forced vital capacity). A ratio of FEV_1/FVC <70% is indicative of obstructive airways disease. As with PEFR, this ratio is *episodically* low in asthmatic individuals.

Chest radiograph

A chest radiograph is normal in most asthmatic individuals. However, during an acute asthma attack, the chest may appear hyperexpanded due to air trapping in the obstructed airways. Mucous gland hypersecretion may cause mucus plugging that can cause collapse of a lobe or segment of lung, which appears as increased shadowing in the affected area of the lung field.

Diagnosis

Asthma is diagnosed by a *history suggestive of asthma* plus either:

- >15% increase in FEV_1 or PEFR following use of a bronchodilator, or
- >15% variability in PEFR during home monitoring, i.e. demonstration of morning dipping.

Management

The British Thoracic Society Guidelines (2003)[1] give a five-step method for the management of asthma. The patient is started at Step 1 and moved to other steps until control of asthma symptoms is achieved:

- *Step 1:* short-acting β_2-agonist inhaler for bronchodilatation (e.g. salbutamol) used when needed only.
- *Step 2:* Step 1 + low-dose inhaled corticosteroid (200–800 μg/day) to suppress the inflammatory response (e.g. beclometasone) used regularly.
- *Step 3:* Step 2 + long-acting β_2-agonist inhaler (e.g. salmeterol) used regularly. If there is no response to long-acting β_2-agonist inhaler, stop it and try another agent, such as slow-release theophylline or a leukotriene antagonist (e.g. montelukast).
- *Step 4:* Step 3 + high-dose inhaled steroid (up to 2000 μg) used regularly. Another agent such as slow-release theophylline, a leukotriene antagonist (e.g. montelukast) or oral slow-release β_2-agonist may be tried.
- *Step 5:* Step 4 + oral steroids used regularly.

5-lipoxygenase inhibitors or recombinant humanized monoclonal anti-IgE antibody are becoming available for use.

Acute severe asthma (status asthmaticus)

This is a life-threatening condition.

Features of an acute severe attack of asthma
- Unable to speak in full sentences.
- Pulse rate >110/min.
- PEFR <50% of patient's normal value.

Features of a life-threatening attack of asthma
- Unable to speak.
- Silent chest: breath sounds not audible on auscultation with stethoscope.
- PEFR <33% of patient's normal value.
- Central cyanosis.

Management
- *PEFR measurement.*
- *Arterial blood gas measurement:* the PaO_2 (partial pressure of oxygen) may be low, indicating hypoxia. In extreme cases, the $PaCO_2$ (partial pressure of carbon dioxide) may be high and the pH may be low.
- *Oxygen* via mask (at high concentration).
- *Salbutamol* (β_2 agonist) via nebulizer every 15–30 min.
- *Steroids:* intravenous hydrocortisone 200 mg or oral prednisone 30–40 mg.
- If symptoms persist, try:
  - ipratropium bromide (anticholinergic)
  - IV salbutamol.

Caution
Exhaustion, drowsiness, worsening hypoxia (PaO_2 <8 kPa, falling), hypercapnoea ($PaCO_2$ >6 kPa, rising) and acidosis are signs of imminent respiratory arrest and, if these develop, immediately refer to ITU for mechanical ventilation.

Dental aspects

- Elective dental care should be deferred in severe asthmatics.
- Asthmatic patients should bring their usual medication with them and use them if an attack is impending.
- Avoid drugs that may precipitate an attack, particularly aspirin, or non-steroidal anti-inflammatory drugs (NSAIDs).
- Local anaesthesia (LA) is best used for dental treatment.
- Avoid LA solutions containing vasoconstrictors, since occasional patients react to the sulphites present in preservatives.
- Allergy to penicillin may be more frequent.
- Leukotriene-modifying drugs may prolong the INR (international normalized ratio), causing a bleeding tendency.
- Systemic corticosteroid treatment brings with it the need for steroid cover (see chapter on adrenal disorders).
- Corticosteroid inhalers occasionally cause oral or pharyngeal thrush.

Reference

1. The British Thoracic Society. The BTS/SIGN British guidance on the management of asthma. *Thorax* 2003; 58: Supplement I.

Five facts

1. Asthma is reversible airways obstruction caused by bronchospasm.
2. Asthma is an allergic, IgE-mediated type I hypersensitivity reaction.
3. Most cases of asthma are found in atopic individuals in conjunction with other allergic conditions, e.g. eczema, hayfever.
4. PEFR is a simple bedside test for the diagnosis of airflow obstruction during an asthma attack.
5. An acute asthma attack should be treated initially with high-flow oxygen, salbutamol nebulizers and IV hydrocortisone.

Back pain

Acute back pain

Acute back pain with no associated neurological disturbance after an injury is common, and it is the easiest type of back pain to diagnose. It is treated initially with rest and non-steroidal anti-inflammatory drugs (NSAIDs) for their combined anti-inflammatory and analgesic roles. It is important not to allow the large back muscles (erector spinae and the like) to remain in spasm, as this can provoke chronic back pain, and hence, after a couple of days rest, limited movement should be commenced.

Chronic back pain

Chronic back pain is one of the most common and troublesome of complaints. More working hours are lost to chronic back pain than any other single condition in the UK. Its exact diagnosis can be difficult, but a careful history and examination, followed by a multidisciplinary approach to management can be extremely rewarding.

In assessing such patients it is important to address three questions:

1. Is there no obvious mechanical cause but rather clear cut spinal pathology? If yes, this includes vertebral infections, spinal tumours, ankylosing spondylitis, polyarthritis, Paget's disease and primary neurological conditions.
2. Is the pain associated with nerve root (radicular) symptoms? If yes, the commonest cause is a prolapsed intervertebral disc.
3. Is there a mechanical cause? If yes, this includes osteoporotic wedge fractures, spondylolisthesis, osteoarthritis and Scheuermann's disease.

In some patients it is impossible to identify an exact cause, and it is these patients that are notoriously difficult to manage.

History and examination

It is said that 80% of medical diagnoses can be made from the history alone, and this is certainly true of chronic back pain.

A history asking about all the characteristics of pain (e.g. site, character, nature, relieving and aggravating factors) is vital. It is crucial to ask about radicular symptoms, such as the sharp, knife-like pain radiating down the legs typical of nerve root involvement. If the pain radiates below the knee to the ankle or foot, this is suggestive of nerve compression pain, and not osteoarthritis of the hip, in which the pain can radiate down to the knee but not beyond. Motor involvement should be enquired about along with disturbances in gait, balance, bowel or bladder function, raising suspicion of nerve involvement. A general systems enquiry may raise the possibility of tuberculosis or malignancy.

Examination of the spine should involve palpation of the vertebral spines, the surrounding musculature, the interspinous spaces, as well as a peripheral neurological examination assessing sensation, and muscle:

1. tone
2. power
3. reflexes
4. co-ordination.

Attention should be paid to delineating abnormalities in specific dermatomes and myotomes, so that any nerve lesion can be localized.

If the diagnosis cannot be made without investigations – e.g. radiograph, bone scan, magnetic resonance imaging (MRI) – the patient should be referred for an orthopaedic opinion.

Causes of chronic back pain

Scoliosis
Scoliosis is a *lateral* curvature of the spine, which may be due to an alteration in vertebral shape and mobility (structural scoliosis) or may occur with normal vertebrae (non-structural scoliosis).

Structural scoliosis is seen with poliomyelitis, cerebral palsy, spina bifida, syringomyelia, rickets, and Marfan syndrome among others, but in most cases the cause is unknown (idiopathic). Structural scoliosis always needs investigating to rule out the serious causes mentioned.

Non-structural scoliosis can be a compensatory response due to tilting of the pelvis from shortening of one leg, but is most commonly a postural phenomenon seen in adolescent girls. Postural scoliosis is remedied with conservative measures, such as adopting a straight posture, and most girls grow out of it by adulthood.

Kyphosis
Kyphosis is a *forward* curvature of the spine, causing the classic dowager's hump appearance of the famous Hunchback of Notre Dame. Again, this may result from serious causes like poliomyelitis, muscular dystrophy, ankylosing spondylitis, senile kyphosis, Paget's disease, tuberculosis, fractures and tumours, or it can be postural. In adults, the commonest tumour is a metastatic deposit, whereas in children it is usually a benign tumour.

Scheuermann's disease
This condition is characterized by the anterior parts of the vertebrae growing slower than the posterior parts (anterior wedging), leading to kyphosis, impaired mobility and secondary osteoarthritis.

Ankylosing spondylitis
In ankylosing spondylitis, there is progressive ossification of the joints of the spine. It almost invariably involves the sacroiliac joints and back, and may involve the costovertebral joints, limiting chest expansion and ventilation. If it involves the cervical spine, then neck stiffness will be seen; endotracheal intubation and other airway securing procedures in these patients can lead to snapping of the cervical vertebrae with consequent paralysis if not performed with extreme caution.

The cause is unknown but it appears most commonly in young and middle-aged men with a positive family history. Classically, patients have a raised erythrocyte sedimentation rate (ESR), are positive for HLA-B27, but negative for rheumatoid factor. They may also have anaemia, muscle wasting and weight loss.

Senile kyphosis
As people become elderly, they become progressively stooped and shorter in stature, due to degenerative thinning of the intervertebral discs, sometimes associated with osteoporotic wedging of the vertebrae.

Paget's disease
Paget's disease typically affects the pelvis and is unusual in the spine. However, if it does occur, it can lead to spinal cord problems.

Tuberculosis
Bone and joint tuberculosis (TB) is uncommon in the UK but its incidence is increasing along with other types of TB. This is because of the development of drug-resistant strains, the rise of HIV and an increasing immigrant population. Spinal TB usually progresses slowly, with aching chronic back pain. Later, the anterior parts of the vertebrae collapse and the spine becomes angulated. A TB spinal abscess can form and track distally, causing compression of the spinal cord with consequent limb weakness or paralysis. Plain radiographs, computed tomography (CT) and MRI may all help in assessing the extent of damage, and CT-guided needle drainage may resolve any neurological compromise.

Metastases
Metastases, the commonest tumours in adult spines, are particularly seen in the elderly. Some primary neoplasms are more likely to metastasize to the spine than others – adenocarcinoma of the prostate is probably the most notorious.

Radiographs and bone scans are usually diagnostic, and radiotherapy may provide palliation.

Spondylolysis and spondylolisthesis
When standing upright there is a tendency for the body of the fifth lumbar vertebra (L5) to slip forwards on the top of the sacrum as the plane of the L5–S1 disc slopes downwards anteriorly. This is usually prevented by the articular processes (facet joints). However, a defect or fracture of L5 anterior to its inferior articular process may allow this slip to occur. Before a slip the condition is known as spondylolysis and after the slip it is called spondylolisthesis. Commonly, these conditions present as low back pain that radiates into the buttocks.

Cauda equina syndrome
The cauda equina is the 'horse's tail'-like structure of nerve roots exiting the end of the spinal cord to supply the lower limbs and pelvis. Compression of the nerve roots here results in lower limb weakness, bilateral sciatica (radicular pain down both legs), loss of perianal sensation and anal tone and disturbance of bowel and bladder function (typically double incontinence). Such signs should prompt immediate treatment with high-dose corticosteroids, urgent MRI to confirm the diagnosis and then

surgical decompression. If these measures are not instituted within 6 hours, then the patient is at high risk for permanent paralysis and incontinence.

Osteoarthritis
Primary osteoarthritis (OA) of the spine is extremely common, as the spine bears the weight of the body and is thus subject to considerable wear and tear. Typically, OA affects many spinal levels and the classical features of OA (disc degeneration, anterior and posterior lipping of the vertebrae and narrowing of the facet joints) are present.

Rheumatoid arthritis
Rheumatoid arthritis (RA) can affect the spine but is far commoner at other sites (see chapter on arthritis). If RA affects the neck, then endotracheal intubation can be very difficult due to the stiff cervical spine.

Spina bifida
In spina bifida there is congenital non-fusion of the posterior parts of the spine, with possible herniation of the spinal cord. Depending on the severity of the defect and the degree of resulting herniation, the patient may be symptom-free (as in spina bifida occulta, where the only obvious abnormality is a tuft of hair overlying the bifid segment), or totally paralysed and incontinent.

Spinal stenosis
A decrease in the sagittal diameter of the spinal canal can give rise to lower limb pain and paraesthesiae with exercise (so-called neurogenic claudication). By bending forwards when the pain appears, the patient opens up his spinal canal, thus reducing compression on the cord with subsequent relief of symptoms. When you walk up a hill or up stairs you do so with your spine bent forward, and thus neurological claudicants get better walking upwards and worse when going down stairs. This is in contrast to patients with peripheral vascular disease, whose intermittent claudication has the reverse characteristics.

Spinal stenosis can be caused by OA, spondylolisthesis, Paget's disease, fracture, spinal surgery and dwarfism. CT and MRI can show the decreased spaces within the spinal canal for neurological structures.

Prolapsed intervertebral disc
Each intervertebral disc contains a central semi-liquid material called the nucleus pulposus contained within the annulus. If a tear in the annulus occurs (usually from injury), then the nucleus pulposus may protrude out of the disc – a so-called prolapsed intervertebral disc. This causes acute back pain. Spinal nerves lie in posterolateral relation to the intervertebral discs and can therefore also be compressed by such prolapses – with neurological sequelae.

The discs that most commonly prolapse are L5/S1, then L4/L5, and then L3/L4, causing compression of spinal nerves S1, L5 and L4, respectively. S1 compression typically causes loss of sensation over the dorsal aspect of the little toe on the side of disc prolapse, decreased power in hallux plantarflexion and a diminished ankle jerk. L5 compression typically causes anaesthesia over the dorsal aspect of the hallux or lateral aspect of the shin and decreased hallux dorsiflexion. L4 compression typically causes decreased sensation over the medial aspect of the shin, weakened knee extension and a diminished knee jerk. With large central prolapses, the cauda equina can be involved, leading to cauda equina syndrome.

In the long term, prolapsed intervertebral discs can cause narrowing of the disc spaces and subsequent secondary osteoarthritis, causing chronic back pain.

Mechanical back pain

This diagnosis should never be made until all other causes are excluded by an orthopaedic surgeon. Sadly, a number of patients have lingering chronic back pain of no obvious cause and are hampered by this for the rest of their lives. A multi-disciplinary approach involving orthopaedic surgeons, physiotherapists and, occasionally, pain specialists is required.

Coccydynia

Coccydynia is chronic pain in the 'tail end'. Often it is preceded by a fall, and occasionally radiographs show a coccygeal fracture. Chronic pain on seating or defaecation may last several months, but usually resolves spontaneously with analgesia and psychological support. Surgery to remove the coccyx is a last resort and is rarely successful.

Dental aspects

Endotracheal intubation and other airway-securing procedures in patients with ankylosing spondylitis or rheumatoid arthritis can lead to paralysis if not performed with extreme caution.

Five facts

1. Chronic back pain is a major cause of morbidity in the community.
2. Cauda equina syndrome is an emergency and requires immediate treatment, often with steroids and/or surgical decompression.
3. Prolapsed intervertebral disc is often associated with radicular pain.
4. Spina bifida can result in paralysis, and loss of bowel and bladder control.
5. Extreme caution is needed in performing endotracheal intubation in patients with ankylosing spondylitis and rheumatoid arthritis.

Bleeding tendency

Haemostasis is the physical cessation of bleeding. It involves:

1. vascular injury with exposure of subendothelial tissue factor and collagen
2. vasoconstriction
3. platelet aggregation at the site of injury (platelet plug)
4. activation of the clotting cascade
5. platelet plug stabilized with fibrin
6. fibrinolysis and vasodilatation
7. homeostatic mechanisms to achieve a balance between haemostasis and fibrinolysis.

Various prothrombotic (e.g. von Willebrand factor, platelet activating factor) and antithrombotic (e.g. nitric oxide, tissue plasminogen activator) factors are involved in the above response.

The clotting cascade involves a variety of coagulation factors and two distinct pathways (extrinsic and intrinsic) that come together as the final common pathway and result in the formation of cross-linked fibrin that stabilizes the platelet plug to form a clot. Heparin exerts its antithrombotic effect by inhibiting the intrinsic pathway, and warfarin works by inhibiting the extrinsic pathway. The activated partial thromboplastin time (APTT) is a measure of intrinsic function and is therefore increased by heparin therapy. The prothrombin time (PT) and the international normalized ratio (INR) are measures of extrinsic function and are increased by warfarin.

Disorders of the blood vessel wall, platelets or the coagulation pathway may all lead to a bleeding tendency. *Thus, a full blood count (FBC, to measure number of platelets) and clotting profile (to measure PT, APTT and fibrinogen) will detect the vast majority of coagulopathies.* By far the most common causes of a bleeding tendency are drugs (e.g. warfarin, aspirin and non-steroidal anti-inflammatory drugs (NSAIDs)), liver failure and renal failure.

Disorders of blood vessel wall

Bleeding is only rarely due to blood vessel defects. *Hereditary haemorrhagic telangiectasia* is a rare, autosomal dominant disorder characterized by disordered blood vessel structure. In the skin, respiratory and gastrointestinal tracts, abnormal telangiectasia (dilated capillaries) may form and are susceptible to recurrent bleeding.

Disorders of platelet function

If the platelet count drops below 50×10^9/L (normal 150–400 $\times 10^9$/L), then spontaneous bleeding can occur. Thrombocytopenia (low platelets) may be caused by decreased production, increased destruction or sequestration. In addition, platelet function itself may be inhibited in the absence of thrombocytopenia.

Decreased megakaryocyte production/maturation
- Bone marrow aplasia is usually idiopathic, but viruses such as human parvovirus B19 and drugs such as cytotoxics may be causal factors.

- Bone marrow suppression can be caused by leukaemia, myeloma or carcinoma.
- Inadequate maturation of platelet precursors (megakaryocytes) can be caused by vitamin B_{12} or folate deficiency.

Increased platelet destruction
- Viral infections such as Epstein–Barr virus (EBV) and HIV damage platelets.
- *Idiopathic thrombocytopenic purpura* (ITP) is an autoimmune disorder which causes platelet destruction.
- *Haemolytic uraemic syndrome* (HUS) is caused by small vessel wall damage, which leads to fibrin and platelet deposition (microangiopathic haemolytic anaemia, MAHA), and predominantly affects the kidneys. *Escherichia coli* O157 gastroenteritis may cause HUS in children.
- *Thrombotic thrombocytopenic purpura* (TTP) is similar to HUS but tends to affect the brain. *E. coli* O157 gastroenteritis is more commonly associated with TTP in adults.
- *Disseminated intravascular coagulopathy* (DIC; see below) leads to consumption of platelets.

Sequestration of platelets
This condition occurs in splenomegaly, and may therefore be caused by a host of disorders including the following:

- portal hypertension, e.g. cirrhosis
- haematological disorders, e.g. myeloproliferative disorders
- infections, e.g. malaria, leishmaniasis, Epstein–Barr virus
- storage disorders, e.g. Gaucher's disease, Niemann–Pick disease
- inflammatory disorders, e.g. SLE (systemic lupus erythematosus), Felty's syndrome.

Platelets can be replaced or supplemented by platelet transfusions, but sequestration of transfused platelets is very rapid.

Impairment of platelet function

Renal failure
Renal failure leads to high serum levels of urea, which directly inhibit platelet function and thrombocytopenia. Desmopressin (DDAVP) may be used to treat mild bleeding episodes. In severe bleeding, cryoprecipitate or platelet transfusion may be required.

Drugs
Platelet cyclo-oxygenase (COX) is an enzyme which catalyses the production of thromboxane A_2 from arachidonic acid. Thromboxane A_2 is an important factor in platelet aggregation during thrombus formation.

Aspirin is an irreversible inhibitor of COX, and thus leads to a bleeding tendency (as do other NSAIDs).

Disorders of blood coagulation

Congenital disorders

von Willebrand's disease

von Willebrand's disease is the most common inherited bleeding disorder, affecting 1 in 1000 individuals. Most cases are autosomal dominant. It is caused by deficiency of von Willebrand factor (vWF), a protein synthesized by both platelets and the endothelial cells of blood vessels. vWF has two main functions: as a carrier protein for factor VIII, and to aid platelet adhesion to damaged endothelium.

Clinical features
von Willebrand's disease is principally a disease of platelet function, but also affects clotting. Bruising, nosebleeds (epistaxis) and prolonged bleeding during surgical procedures are the common complaints. Menorrhagia and gastrointestinal haemorrhage are also common.

Investigations
The bleeding time is prolonged and vWF levels are reduced. However, factor VIII levels are sufficient to provide a normal APTT, and the PT is also normal.

Management
In mild bleeding, DDAVP may be used to acutely increase the vWF levels. In more severe cases, cryoprecipitate or vWF concentrate may be needed.

Haemophilia A

Haemophilia A affects 1 in 10 000 males and is caused by mutations in the blood clotting factor VIII gene, leading to factor VIII deficiency. It has X-linked inheritance; therefore, all males with the gene are affected, and all women with the gene are carriers. The severity of the disease depends on the levels of functioning factor VIII:

- *Severe disease* produces frequent bleeding after minor trauma: <1% (of normal levels of) factor VIII.
- *Moderate disease* produces less frequent bleeding: 1–5% factor VIII.
- *Mild disease* gives persistent bleeding usually only after significant trauma: 5–25% factor VIII.

Clinical features
Bleeding may be deep into tissues or spaces such as the joints or in almost any site of the body:

- *Haemarthrosis* (bleeding into joints) may occur without any significant trauma in severe disease. Acute features include joint pain, swelling and decreased range of movement. Repeated episodes lead to joint deformity and osteoarthrosis.
- *Muscle haematoma* presents with pain and swelling. The haematoma can enlarge to compress surrounding structures such as nerves and arteries. Fibrosis may occur, and causes permanent shortening of the muscle and thus limitation of movement of the limb.
- *Intracranial haemorrhage* is potentially life-threatening.

Investigations
Factor VIII assay will show markedly reduced levels of factor VIII. APTT is prolonged but PT is normal.

Management
Pooled factor VIII from donor serum is used prophylactically before surgery to treat bleeding episodes. During surgery, factor VIII levels may need to be maintained to prevent sustained intra- and post-operative haemorrhage. This is usually done with a factor VIII concentrate or DDAVP infusion. The most serious complication of factor VIII infusion is the transmission of blood-borne viral infections, such as hepatitis B, hepatitis C and HIV infection. Thus, most haemophiliac adults are HCV positive, and most have been exposed to HBV (a proportion of which are carriers). Recombinant factor VIII is now used to avoid this complication.

Haemophilia B (Christmas disease)
Haemophilia B is clinically identical to haemophilia A, but is 10 times less common. Haemophilia B is an X-linked disorder caused by mutations in the factor IX gene which lead to factor IX deficiency. The factor IX levels are low, and APTT is prolonged with a normal PT. Treatment is with factor IX concentrate.

Acquired disorders

Liver disease
The liver is the major site of synthesis of vitamin K-dependent clotting factors such as II, VII, IX, X and fibrinogen. In liver disease, synthesis is reduced, which leads to prolongation of the PT.

Patients with liver failure may have oesophageal varices associated with portal hypertension, and bleeding from these varices in the presence of clotting factor deficiency is an extremely serious complication associated with a high mortality.

Treatment with regular high-dose vitamin K increases rates of synthesis of these clotting factors. During episodes of bleeding, fresh frozen plasma (FFP) may be needed to supplement levels of these clotting factors.

Drugs

Warfarin
Warfarin prolongs the PT and the INR by inhibiting the activation of clotting factors II, VII, IX and X by vitamin K. The advantage of warfarin is that it is an orally administered drug, and is therefore suitable for home administration. It takes 2–3 days for the anticoagulant effects to fully occur and several days for its effects to wear off. INR monitoring must regularly be performed on all patients so that the dose of warfarin may be adjusted appropriately.

Heparin
Unfractionated heparin prolongs the APTT by potentiating antithrombin III, which inhibits the activation of clotting factors II, IX, X and XI. It is given via intravenous

infusion, with the dose titrated according to the APTT. The half-life of unfraction-ated heparin is only 1 hour, making it useful where rapid normalization of anticoag-ulation is required, e.g. prior to surgery. If more rapid reversal of heparin anticoagulation is needed, protamine may be used. Low molecular weight heparin (LMWH) acts more specifically on inhibition of factor X activation. The APTT is therefore normal. Factor Xa assay may be used to monitor the anticoagulant effect of LMWH, but this is not routinely required.

Disseminated intravascular coagulopathy (DIC)

DIC is the uncontrolled consumption of clotting factors and intravascular deposition (and therefore depletion in circulating blood) of platelets and fibrin, to produce serious coagulopathy and thrombocytopenia. It may be caused by many conditions, including sepsis, trauma, adenocarcinoma, acute myeloid leukaemia and amniotic fluid embolus.

In DIC, levels of fibrinogen are low (due to consumption of fibrin) and fibrin degra-dation products are high. The PT, APTT and bleeding time are all raised.

The deposition of platelets and fibrin in small blood vessels associated with DIC produces *microangiopathic haemolytic anaemia* (MAHA), because it causes damage to erythrocytes (haemolysis) and damage to the small blood vessels (microangiopathy). HUS and TTP (see section on increased platelet destruction) are pathologically less severe forms of DIC, and many of their clinical features are due to microangiopathy affecting either the kidney (as in HUS) or the brain (as in TTP).

Dental aspects

- The common pattern in a bleeding tendency is bleeding from, and purpura of, gingivae and mucous membranes.
- Prolonged bleeding after surgery is one of the most common signs of haemor-rhagic disease and may amount to a haemorrhagic emergency. It is sometimes the way by which the disease is first recognized.
- Replacement therapy is required before surgery, and ideally all necessary surgery (and other dental treatment) should be performed at one operation.
- Intraligamentary or intraosseous local anaesthetic injections are safe.
- Local anaesthetic regional blocks, lingual infiltrations or injections into the floor of the mouth must not be used unless replacement therapy is being given, because of the risk of haemorrhage into fascial spaces of the neck hazarding the airway and becoming life-threatening.
- Intramuscular injections of drugs should be avoided unless replacement therapy is being given, as they can cause large haematomas.
- The bleeding tendency can be aggravated by analgesics. It may also be aggra-vated by other factors such as liver damage after hepatitis, HIV disease, throm-bocytopenia, and drugs such as protease inhibitors and aspirin or other NSAIDs. Acetaminophen (paracetamol), codeine and COX-2 inhibitors are safer.

Five facts

1. Bleeding tendency is produced by disorders of coagulation, platelet function and the blood vessel wall.
2. By far the most common causes of bleeding tendency are drugs (such as warfarin, aspirin and NSAIDs), renal failure and liver failure.
3. A full blood count (to measure number of platelets) and clotting profile (to measure PT, APTT and fibrinogen) will detect the vast majority of coagulopathies.
4. Acetaminophen (paracetamol) and codeine are safer types of analgesia in a patient with bleeding tendency.
5. Local anaesthetic regional blocks, lingual infiltrations, injections into the floor of the mouth and intramuscular injections must *not* be used in bleeding tendency unless replacement therapy is being given.

Breast cancer

Epidemiology

Breast cancer affects roughly 1 in 10 women in the developed world and is the commonest cause of death in women aged 40–50. The incidence of breast cancer increases with increasing age (rare before age 30), although death rates peak at 40–50 years and then drop off, probably because older women die of other causes before breast cancer becomes significant. Breast cancer is more common in Caucasian women than in women of African or Asian descent.

Risk factors

Personal history of breast cancer
Women who have had breast cancer face a greater risk of getting cancer in the other breast.

Family history
A woman's risk of developing breast cancer rises if her mother, sister or daughter has had breast cancer, especially at a young age.

Genetics
Changes in certain genes (BRCA1, BRCA2 and others) increase the risk of breast cancer.

Histological changes
Having a diagnosis of atypical hyperplasia or lobular carcinoma in situ (LCIS) are risk factors for developing cancer.

Other factors associated with a higher risk for breast cancer

Oestrogen
The longer a woman is exposed to oestrogen, the more likely she is to develop breast cancer. The oral contraceptive pill (OCP) and hormone replacement therapy (HRT) if used in the long term are risk factors.

Late childbearing
Women who have their first child late (after about age 30) have a greater chance of developing breast cancer.

Breast density
Cancer is more likely to occur in breasts that have a great deal of lobular and ductal tissue.

Radiation therapy
There is a higher risk, especially in patients treated with radiation for Hodgkin's disease.

Alcohol
There is a slightly higher risk of breast cancer among women who drink alcohol.

Fat
A fatty diet appears to confer a greater risk of breast cancer.

Smoking
Whether smoking is a risk factor is controversial, with much conflicting evidence having been reported in recent years.

Pathology

Breast carcinoma may be either derived from ductal (90%) or lobular (10%) epithelium. Pre-invasive *in situ* forms of tumour exist but the majority are invasive.

Ductal carcinoma can be classified into non-specific invasive ductal type (the vast majority) and other types (medullary, tubular, mucoid and papillary), which generally have a better prognosis. Paget's disease is an intra-epithelial ductal carcinoma.

Lobular carcinoma may be invasive or *in situ*, when it is often bilateral.

Breast carcinomas, as is typical of most solid malignancies, spread via four main routes:

1. Direct extension into skin, causing dimpling and an orange-peel (peau d'orange) appearance, nipple retraction and ulceration, and into muscle and the chest wall.
2. The lymphatic route into dermal lymphatics, and into axillary and internal thoracic lymph nodes.
3. The haematogenous route to the lungs, liver and bones (at sites of red bone marrow, i.e. skull, vertebrae, pelvis, sternum, ribs, upper humerus and upper femur) and, less commonly, to the brain, ovaries and adrenal glands.
4. The trans-coelomic route to the pleural cavity, causing pleural effusions, and to the peritoneal cavity, causing effusions (ascites).

Clinical features

Features include a painless lump in the breast, breast pain (mastalgia), nipple changes (such as retraction or bloody discharge) or symptoms secondary to metastases (such as back pain, pathological fracture pain or shortness of breath from pleural effusions or lung metastases). Early breast cancer does *not* usually cause pain.

Investigations and staging

Any patient with a suspicious breast lump should be referred to a breast surgeon immediately. Such patients are usually seen in a '*triple assessment clinic*' where clinical history and examination, imaging and biopsy are all performed. Imaging is either by mammography or, in younger patients whose breasts are too dense to visualize well with mammography, by ultrasonography.

A tissue diagnosis is obtained either by fine needle aspiration cytology (FNAC) or core-cut biopsy (if FNAC yields insufficient tissue for diagnosis). Sometimes a sample of breast tissue is checked for the human epidermal growth factor receptor-2 or HER-2 gene that is associated with a higher risk of cancer recurrence.

The tumour is then staged using chest radiography, bone scanning, liver ultrasound and a full blood count (anaemia and leucopenia suggest widespread bone marrow involvement). Breast carcinomas are usually staged in the standard TNM (**T**umour, **N**odes, **M**etastasis) system devised by the American Joint Committee for Cancer (AJCC). A simpler staging system devised in Manchester, UK, stages in four groups:

- Stage 1: lump confined to the breast with no features of more advanced disease.
- Stage 2: lump confined to the breast, but with enlarged, mobile axillary lymph nodes.
- Stage 3: lump confined to the breast but the tumour and/or nodes are fixed.
- Stage 4: distant metastases are present.

Management

Stages 1 and 2 tumours are usually treated by 'curative' surgery, whereas those in stages 3 and 4 are only suitable for palliative treatment. The results from conservative surgical approaches are as good as those achieved by the radical mastectomy pioneered by William Halsted at Johns Hopkins Hospital in Baltimore, USA.

Hence most surgeons perform their curative surgery with a wide local excision (WLE), having at least a 1 cm margin, together with axillary lymph node sampling (>3 nodes) or clearance (removing all the axillary nodes). Some breast surgeons are performing *sentinel node biopsy* where just one axillary node, the usual node of first spread of the tumour, is removed to check for spread.

Postoperatively, radiotherapy may be given. In advanced stage 2 disease with extensive lymph node involvement there may also be a role for adjuvant (postoperative) chemotherapy or hormonal therapy, and clinical trials investigating this are also underway.

If, on histopathological analysis of the WLE, there is tumour at the excision margins, a further excision or simple mastectomy is performed.

Palliative treatment for stages 3 and 4 usually consists of surgical debulking of the primary lesion if it is fungating and ulcerative, and local radiotherapy to any painful metastatic deposits.

Antioestrogens such as tamoxifen are used to treat widespread metastases (adjuvant therapy). Patients who fail to respond to tamoxifen can be offered second-line agents, and are best seen by an oncologist. Tamoxifen can increase the risk of uterine cancer and strokes; anastrozole is a safer alternative. Trastuzumab is a monoclonal antibody that targets breast cancer cells that have an excess of HER-2 and may be given alone or along with chemotherapy.

Prognosis

As is true of most malignancies, the stage and grade of tumours are important in predicting prognosis. Stage 1 tumours have a 5-year survival rate of around 80%, dropping to 50% at 10 years. Stage 2 lesions have a 5-year survival of around 50%, with the more advanced stages having survival rates of <10% at 5 years. Poorly differentiated tumours have a worse prognosis than well differentiated ones.

Various models exist in predicting prognosis for an individual patient. The most commonly used model is the Nottingham Prognostic Index (NPI), which considers stage, grade and size of tumour.

Screening

Mortality can be reduced by up to 30% in women who attend screening. In 1986 the Forest Report looked at the New York and Swedish screening programmes and made screening recommendations for UK women. These recommendations were that women between 50 and 65 years old should be invited every 3 years for a single oblique mammogram (although in practice most breast units perform two views on the first screening visit). About 60 cancers per 10 000 attendees are detected in the UK screening programme.

Male breast cancer

Male breast cancer accounts for <1% of all cases of breast cancer. It presents in the same way as the female equivalent and is managed similarly. However, due to the proximity of the male breast to the chest wall, cancer usually presents with more locally advanced disease, leading to a poorer prognosis in general.

Dental aspects

Metastases from breast cancer occasionally affect the jaws and are most typically seen in the premolar/molar region of the mandible, where there is haematopoietic bone marrow. Pain or neuropathy with paraesthesia or hypoaesthesia may result.

Five facts

1. Breast cancer affects roughly 1 in 10 women in the Western world.
2. Patients should be referred for 'triple assessment', i.e. clinical examination, imaging and biopsy.
3. Conservative surgical approaches with or without immediate breast reconstruction are more popular than radical mastectomy.
4. Less than 1% of all cases of breast cancer occur in men.
5. Breast cancer can metastasize to the mandible.

Chronic obstructive pulmonary disease

Chronic obstructive pulmonary disease (COPD) represents the spectrum of lung disease that includes chronic bronchitis and emphysema, previously called chronic obstructive airways disease, and is characterized by chronic, non-reversible airways obstruction. *Chronic bronchitis* is defined as a cough on most days, for at least 3 consecutive months per year, for at least 2 years. *Emphysema* is defined as the destruction and enlargement of airways distal to the terminal bronchioles. It is therefore a pathological rather than a clinical diagnosis.

Clinical features

Common features of COPD include:

- *chronic cough* productive of purulent sputum
- *recurrent chest infections*
- wheeze
- shortness of breath.

In advanced COPD, common clinical signs include:

- *cyanosis* (peripheral or central)
- *chest hyperexpansion* (barrel chest)
- *tracheal tug* (downward descent of the trachea in inspiration)
- *intercostal recession* (pulling in of the skin between the ribs on inspiration)
- *pursed lip breathing* – designed to increase intrathoracic pressure in expiration, thus preventing airways collapse
- *cor pulmonale* (right-sided heart failure) may occur in advanced COPD, with a raised jugular venous pressure (JVP), pitting ankle oedema and a right ventricular heave.

Pathology

By far the commonest cause of COPD is smoking, which causes chronic inflammation of the airways.

Chronic bronchitis
Chronic inflammation in the bronchi leads to goblet cell hyperplasia, leading to mucus hypersecretion and thus chronic cough and sputum production. Damage to the airway cilia impairs clearance of secretions, and promotes infection.

Emphysema
Smoking promotes macrophage-mediated proteinases, causing destruction of the elastic component of the small airways, which therefore become dilated and more collapsible in expiration. This leads to airways obstruction. Furthermore, the surface area of epithelium involved in gas exchange is reduced, which causes hypoxia.

Destruction of the lung parenchyma leads to modification of the pulmonary vasculature and this may eventually lead to pulmonary hypertension and subsequent cor pulmonale (right-sided heart failure).

In most patients with emphysema there is also an element of bronchoconstriction, but this only accounts for less than 15% of airways obstruction. This is in contrast to asthma, where virtually all the obstruction is from bronchoconstriction.

Alpha₁-antitrypsin deficiency

Alpha$_1$-antitrypsin deficiency
This rare inherited enzyme deficiency results in uncontrolled proteinase activity, which leads to emphysema, chronic liver disease and cirrhosis in early adulthood.

Type I and type II respiratory failure

Destruction of epithelium involved in gas exchange leads to a reduction in oxygen gas transfer, which causes hypoxia (reduced oxygen).

Hypoxia (PaO_2 <8.6 kPa) with a normal $PaCO_2$ is called type I respiratory failure.

In some patients, hypoventilation may occur, which also leads to hypercapnoea (carbon dioxide retention). Hypoxia (PaO_2 <8.6 kPa) occurring with hypercapnoea ($PaCO_2$ >6 kPa) is called type II respiratory failure. In these patients, an excessively high inspired oxygen concentration reduces the respiratory drive and may even cause respiratory arrest. These patients should therefore only be given a maximum of 28% oxygen (via a Venturi mask).

Investigations

Spirometry

Spirometry provides measurement of FEV_1 (forced expiratory volume in 1 second) and FVC (forced vital capacity). A ratio of FEV_1/FVC <70% of the predicted value, is indicative of obstructive airways disease.

The total lung capacity (TLC) is also estimated. This is increased in COPD, due to gas trapping and the formation of bullae.

The transfer factor is a measure of diffusion capacity across the respiratory epithelium. This becomes reduced in COPD.

Bronchodilator trial

A trial of a β_2-agonist must be used after spirometry is performed to check for significant reversibility in airways obstruction. After the β_2-agonist is given, spirometry is repeated to detect any improvement in FEV_1 (reversibility). If there is >15% (and >200 ml) improvement in FEV_1, the diagnosis is asthma. If reversibility is <15% (or <200 ml), then the diagnosis is COPD. A similar trial should be performed with a 2-week course of high-dose prednisolone.

Arterial blood gas measurement

Arterial blood gas measurement is performed to detect hypoxia and/or hypercapnoea. The extent of hypoxia is important in the assessment of suitability of a patient for long-term oxygen therapy (LTOT) (see below).

Chest radiograph
A chest X-ray may show chest hyperexpansion, as evidenced by enlarged and radiolucent lung fields, and a flattened diaphragm. Bullae appear as large areas with an absence of lung markings.

Sputum culture
A sputum culture is used to detect infection of the airway secretions, which may account for an acute exacerbation of symptoms in COPD. Furthermore, in advanced disease there may be chronic infection with pathogens such as *Haemophilus influenzae*. With the use of repeated courses of antibiotics, antibiotic resistance may rise.

Management

Cessation of smoking
Cessation of smoking is the single most effective treatment of COPD, since it halts the abnormal decline in respiratory function in these patients. Where appropriate, nicotine replacement therapy, or bupropion (amfebutamone) may help.

Oxygen
During an acute exacerbation, oxygen should be given acutely at a maximum concentration of 28% via a Venturi mask. Higher concentrations of oxygen should only be used if arterial blood gases (ABGs) have excluded CO_2 retention (type II respiratory failure).

Bronchodilators
If a bronchodilator trial shows significant reversibility of airflow obstruction, then an inhaled β_2-agonist (e.g. salbutamol) and an inhaled anticholinergic (e.g. ipratropium bromide) should be used. In severe cases of COPD, nebulized bronchodilators, ipratropium bromide, other antimuscarinics (oxitropium), or β_2-agonists, theophylline or low-dose inhaled or systemic corticosteroids are also used.

Oral corticosteroids
Oral corticosteroids are used in high doses (prednisolone 30 mg) to treat acute exacerbations of COPD.

Antibiotics
Antibiotics are used to treat acute exacerbations thought to be infective. Patients typically start to cough copious amounts of purulent (yellow/green) sputum, and may develop haemoptysis. Exacerbations of bronchitis are managed with antibiotics such as amoxicillin, trimethoprim or tetracycline. Immunization against influenza is recommended. Mucolytics such as carbocisteine reduce acute exacerbations by almost one-third. Repeated antibiotic usage and chronic colonization of sputum in some patients may lead to antibiotic resistance, and the need for second- or third-line antibiotic usage.

Long-term oxygen therapy (LTOT)
In severe cases of COPD associated with the development of cor pulmonale, LTOT can reduce pulmonary hypertension, improve quality of life and reduce mortality.

LTOT consists of the delivery of oxygen (2 L/min) via nasal cannulae to patients in their home for at least 15 hours per day. Smoking is an absolute contraindication to LTOT for obvious safety reasons.

Lung reduction surgery
Lung reduction surgery is a treatment for severe COPD used in only a small, selected group of patients.

Transplantation
Single lung or heart–lung transplantation may be performed in end-stage COPD and cor pulmonale that is unresponsive to medical therapy.

Dental aspects

Patients with COPD are best treated in the upright position as they may become breathless if laid flat. It may be difficult to use a rubber dam, as patients may not tolerate the obstruction to breathing. Local anaesthesia is preferred for dental treatment, and patients with COPD should be given relative analgesia only if absolutely necessary, and only in hospital after full preoperative assessment.

Further Reading

The British Thoracic Society Standards of Care Committee. Guidelines on the management of COPD. *Thorax* 1997; 52 (suppl V).

Five facts

1. COPD represents the spectrum of lung disease that includes emphysema and chronic bronchitis.
2. COPD is characterized by predominantly *irreversible* small airways obstruction, in contrast to asthma where it is *reversible*.
3. COPD patients with chronic CO_2 retention must not be given more than 28% oxygen, else impairment of respiratory drive and even respiratory arrest may occur.
4. Exacerbations of COPD should be treated with 28% oxygen (via a Venturi mask), nebulized salbutamol, nebulized ipratropium bromide, oral steroids and antibiotics.
5. Patients with COPD are best treated in the upright position, as they may become breathless if laid flat.

Colorectal cancer

Colorectal carcinoma is the third commonest cancer in men (after lung and prostate) and women (after breast and lung), with a lifetime risk of developing the disease of 5%. Most commonly affected is the distal colon; the rectum in one-third and the sigmoid colon in over one-quarter of cases. In 5% of cases there are multiple tumours (so-called synchronous lesions).

Risk factors for colorectal carcinoma are long-standing ulcerative colitis, pre-existing polyps (adenomas), smoking, a high-fat, low-fibre diet, and a family history. A series of gene alterations leads to adenomas and eventually, in some patients, to carcinoma. Long-term aspirin-taking (or other NSAIDs) lowers the risk of colonic cancer.

In a minority (10% of cases) of colorectal carcinoma, there is a genetic autosomal dominant predisposition, classically presenting in early adulthood in patients with hereditary non-polyposis colorectal carcinoma (HNPCC) or familial adenomatous polyposis (FAP). In HNPCC there are at least four genetic mutations affecting DNA repair mechanisms, whereas in FAP the mutation is of the FAP gene on chromosome 5.

Pathology

Macroscopically, colorectal carcinomas can be polypoid, ulcerating, annular or infiltrative. Microscopically, they are adenocarcinomas (lymphoma, carcinoid and metastases also occur in the large bowel but are generally not included in the term 'colorectal cancer'). Colorectal carcinoma can spread locally into adjacent structures (e.g. small bowel, stomach, duodenum, ureter, bladder, uterus, abdominal wall), via the bloodstream to the liver and lung, via lymphatics to the regional lymph nodes and then to the supraclavicular nodes, and trans-coelomically to produce peritoneal deposits causing ascites.

Clinical features

The manifestations of any malignancy include those produced by the tumour itself, those due to metastases (secondaries) and those due to the general effects of malignancy.

For colorectal carcinoma clinical features include:

- Primary tumour effects – change in bowel habit, passing mucus or blood per rectum, bowel obstruction, perforation causing generalized peritonitis (usually fatal), pericolic abscess or colovesical fistulation. Some patients are detected by the finding of faecal occult blood (FOB) on testing or screening or colonoscopy.
- Effects from metastases – jaundice, ascites, hepatomegaly and chest symptoms.
- General effects of malignancy – weight loss, anorexia and anaemia.

Left-sided tumours tend to be constricting and therefore typically present with bowel obstruction, whereas tumours on the right side, where the stool is not fully formed, are more likely to present with anaemia or weight loss.

It is important for all health care professionals to recognize that any patient with unexplained anaemia or change in bowel habit, including bleeding per rectum, lasting

>4 weeks, should be referred to a gastroenterologist or surgeon for investigation: typically a digital rectal examination and either colonoscopy, barium enema or a computed tomography (CT) scan.

Staging

Colorectal carcinoma may be staged via the universal TNM system, but classically has been staged using a classification developed in the 1920s by a pathologist from St. Mark's Hospital, London called Cuthbert Dukes.

Dukes' A tumours are confined to the mucosa, B tumours go into (B1) or through (B2) the muscularis propria and C tumours have positive regional nodes. Later, a Dukes' D stage was added to represent distant metastases.

Management

Surgical removal of the diseased segment of large bowel along with its regional lymphatics is the standard management of colorectal carcinoma. It is an important point that even in incurable cases with liver metastases, the best palliation is often surgical removal of the primary tumour to relieve or prevent bowel obstruction. In the emergency setting of large bowel obstruction, immediate laparotomy is usually needed, otherwise the patient may perforate and die from generalized peritonitis. With such patients, the risk of sepsis is high and so primary bowel anastomosis is rarely performed and the patient may have a stoma following the immediate operation. In most cases these stomas can be reversed at a later date once the patient has recovered from the bowel obstruction and surgical insult.

Depending on the stage found at histological examination, patients with colorectal carcinoma may require adjuvant chemotherapy and/or radiation treatment. Irinotecan, oxaliplatin, raltitrexed and cetuximab, a monoclonal antibody which targets epidermal growth factor receptor (EGFR), are increasingly used.

Serial monitoring for carcinoembryonic antigen (CEA) in the blood may help detect recurrences.

Prognosis

The 5-year survival is largely dependent on the Dukes' staging of the tumour:

A – 95%
B – 60%
C – 35%
D – <5%

Dental aspects

Familial adenomatous polyposis is a feature of Gardner's syndrome in which multiple exostoses and osteomas of the jaws are seen. These also appear to be more common in patients with non-familial colorectal cancer than in the general population.

Five facts

1. Bowel cancer is the third commonest cancer.
2. Cancer usually arises from pre-existing adenomas (polyps).
3. Aspirin and other NSAID intake reduces the risk of developing bowel cancer.
4. Large bowel obstruction from colorectal carcinoma is an ominous sign.
5. Jaw osteomas are a feature of Gardner's syndrome.

Dermatological conditions

Characteristics of a rash

When faced with a rash, the diagnosis is often unclear, and it may be necessary to describe it to someone on the phone for further advice. In this situation, the student must know how to describe the rash in a methodical way:

- *Distribution*: which parts of the body are affected?
- *Appearance of individual lesions:*
  - Macule: a completely flat lesion.
  - Papule: a raised lesion. A maculopapular rash is the most common type of rash, containing both macules and papules.
  - Vesicle: a small lesion (<5 mm diameter) containing clear fluid.
  - Bulla: a large lesion (>5 mm diameter) containing clear fluid.
  - Pustule: a pus-filled lesion.
  - Plaque: a flat-topped lesion.
- *Colour* of the rash, e.g. erythematous (red), purpuric (purple).
- *Symptoms*, such as pain or itching (pruritis).
- *Additional features*, such as crusting or ulceration.

Acne

Acne vulgaris (acne) affects the majority of teenagers to some degree. However, a minority may continue to be affected by acne in later life. The skin's sebaceous glands, which produce sebum, are associated closely with the hair follicles. Increased sebum production in puberty, and infection with *Propionibacterium acnes,* leads to blockage of the sebaceous ducts and to localized inflammation. Acne is character-ized by papules, pustules, open comedomes (whiteheads) and closed comedomes (blackheads) related to the sebaceous glands. The typical distribution of disease is the face, upper chest and back. The diagnosis is clinical, based on the appearance of the skin.

Management
Mild disease may be treated with topical preparations such as benzoyl peroxide, azelaic acid, or retinoids which act by reducing sebum secretion. Oral antibiotics, e.g. tetracycline, may be used for moderate disease to eradicate *P. acnes* infection. Systemic retinoid therapy, e.g. isotretinoin, is used for severe acne but is highly terato-genic, and therefore must not be used for women who are considering pregnancy.

Psoriasis

Psoriasis is an idiopathic, benign, chronic inflammatory condition with a strong genetic background, that primarily affects skin but may also cause arthritis. It is caused by increased proliferation of keratinocytes in the skin, accompanied by an infiltrate of inflammatory cells.

Clinical features
Skin
Psoriasis is characterized by circular, well demarcated, salmon-pink plaques with a silvery scaly surface. These lesions tend to be on the extensor surfaces of joints, e.g. elbows, the scalp, around the umbilicus and the natal cleft. Other patterns of skin involvement may be less commonly seen. For example, in guttate psoriasis several teardrop-shaped red scaly lesions may appear over the trunk.

Nails
Nail pitting and thickening/separation from the nail bed (onycholysis) may occur.

Joints
Psoriatic arthropathy may occur. The most common type is an asymmetrical small joint arthropathy of the hands. Uncommonly, a severe, disfiguring arthropathy leading to destruction of the small joints of the hands may occur: *arthritis mutilans*.

Diagnosis
The diagnosis is usually made clinically, with a skin biopsy for confirmation in less obvious cases.

Management
- Topical agents such as steroids, retinoids or dithranol (a tar-derived preparation) are all useful in mild disease.
- Ultraviolet light, e.g. PUVA (psoralen plus ultraviolet A), may also be used to treat skin lesions.
- For more severe disease, systemic treatment such as retinoids or immunosuppressive agents may be needed, e.g. methotrexate.

Dental aspects
Oral lesions are rare but there may be a higher prevalence of erythema migrans (geographic tongue), particularly in pustular psoriasis. The temporomandibular joint is involved in up to 60% of patients with psoriatic arthropathy.

Dermatological infections

The infections described in this section are important since they are all spread by direct contact with skin.

Herpes viruses
Herpes simplex virus (HSV) and varicella-zoster virus (VZV) are DNA herpesviruses. After primary infection of the skin or mucosa, HSV and VZV remain dormant in the supplying sensory nerve ganglion to that area. The viruses periodically reactivate to cause infection, particularly during illness, old age or immunosuppression.

HSV causes a localized itchy, painful, vesicular rash with crusting. The typical site for HSV recurrence is around the mouth (cold sore: herpes labialis). HSV may also cause ano-genital ulcers when transmitted by sexual contact.

VZV in a recurrence (zoster or shingles) typically causes unilateral infection of an entire dermatome. For example, infection of the dermatome T4 produces a horizontal strap-like area of vesicles with crusting at the level of the nipple. Itching and pain are typical. In profound immunosuppression (e.g. post-transplant, AIDS), life-threatening systemic VZV infection may occur.

Diagnosis
The diagnosis of these herpesvirus infections is made clinically, but skin scrapings may be analysed with electron microscopy, immunostaining or the polymerase chain reaction (PCR).

Management
Topical treatment with antivirals such as penciclovir or aciclovir is usually used. In severe infections, oral or intravenous aciclovir or valaciclovir may be needed.

Human papillomaviruses
Human papillomaviruses (HPV) are viruses which cause warts and other benign proliferations on the skin and mucosae. Warts are localized, thickened papules and appear mainly on skin predisposed to contact, e.g. hands, face, and as verrucae on the feet (e.g. in swimming pools and saunas). HPV 16 and 18 are sexually transmitted and cause ano-genital warts and predispose to intra-epithelial carcinoma of the vulva and cervical carcinoma.

Diagnosis
The diagnosis is made clinically, but skin scrapings may be analysed with electron microscopy, immunostaining or PCR.

Management
Most warts will regress spontaneously over months to years. However, topical salicylic acid or podophyllin may be used. In refractory cases, cryotherapy is used to freeze off the warts. However, recurrence is common. Imiquimod is an immunostimulatory product that can help treat warts.

Dental aspects
HPV may cause warts or papillomas in the mouth, and some types are associated with some oropharyngeal cancers.

Impetigo
Impetigo is a highly contagious superficial infection caused by *Staphylococcus aureus* or streptococcus. It predominantly affects young children and is associated with poor domestic hygiene. Impetigo is characterized by a vesicular rash which soon crusts to form a yellow, honeycomb-like rash on the face. The diagnosis is clinical, and treatment is with topical fusidic acid or oral flucloxacillin.

Eczema

See the chapter on allergy and anaphylaxis.

Dermatological malignancies

Skin cancer is the most common cancer in both men and women in the developed world and is increasing.

Basal cell carcinoma

Basal cell carcinoma (BCC) is the most common skin cancer. It is predominantly seen in the elderly, affecting sun-exposed areas such as the face and hands. A typical BCC appears as a raised firm lesion with central ulceration and a border that has a typical pink, pearly appearance. It is spread by local extension (rodent ulcer), and metastatic spread is rare.

Treatment is curative with excision, radiotherapy or curettage. Histological examination of the excised tissue is necessary to confirm diagnosis and complete resection of the tumour.

Dental aspects

BCC are rare in the mouth, but multiple skin BCCs are one part of Gorlin's syndrome, when the patient also develops recurrent jaw cysts (odontogenic keratocysts).

Squamous cell carcinoma

Squamous cell carcinoma (SCC) may occur in sun-exposed areas of the skin. Chronic skin inflammation/injury also predisposes to it. Immunosuppression may also lead to SCC, sometimes in association with HPV infection. SCC appears as a hyperkeratotic nodule that develops over several months. SCC tends to spread locally, and may destroy surrounding structures, but metastatic spread is rare. Treatment is the same as for basal cell carcinoma.

Dental aspects

SCC may develop on the lower lip, especially after chronic sun exposure in fair-skinned people, or after organ transplantation.

Malignant melanoma

Melanoma is a neoplasm of melanocytes. It occurs as a result of sun exposure in exposed areas of skin. Melanomas are pigmented, irregular lesions which may bleed and enlarge over months. Unlike SCC and BCC, melanoma can metastasize via the blood after several years. If the tumour has not metastasized, excision biopsy is usually curative. The depth of invasion of the tumour (Breslow thickness) determines the excision margin required for safe removal. Metastatic disease is associated with a very poor prognosis. Chemotherapy is used for metastatic disease, but survival rates are low.

Dental aspects

Melanoma is rare in the mouth but may be seen on the palate.

Five facts

1. Herpes simplex, varicella zoster, impetigo and warts are all infections spread by direct contact.
2. It is therefore important to wear gloves when handling all patients with a rash.
3. Many skin cancers first appear on the sun-exposed areas of the face, e.g. nose, upper lip, ears and scalp.
4. Malignant lesions (in contrast to benign lesions) characteristically increase in size, change shape, bleed and may cause pain or itching.
5. If skin cancer is suspected, an urgent medical opinion should be sought.

Diabetes mellitus

Diabetes mellitus is caused either by insulin deficiency or insulin resistance and is characterized by hyperglycaemia. Diabetes is an extremely common disorder, affecting approximately 150 million people worldwide. The incidence of diabetes is rapidly rising, mostly as an increase in type II diabetes.

Classification

There are two main types of diabetes:

- *Type I* – caused by insulin deficiency   10% of cases
- *Type II* – caused by resistance to insulin   90% of cases

Type I diabetes used to be called insulin-dependent diabetes mellitus (IDDM). Type II diabetes used to be called non insulin-dependent diabetes mellitus (NIDDM). However, this classification should not be used, since some (but not all) type II diabetic patients use insulin injections to control their diabetes, so are by definition insulin-dependent. The distinction based on insulin dependence is therefore false.

Clinical features

About 50% of diabetics are unrecognized. However, common features of diabetes itself include:

- *hyperglycaemia*
- *thirst* and *polyuria* due to glycosuria (glucose in the urine) and subsequent dehydration
- *lethargy*
- *weight loss*.

Complications

Hyperglycaemia leads to vascular disease and a multitude of complications. Diabetes can affect large blood vessels (macrovascular disease) or small blood vessels (microvascular disease). Examples of the effects of macrovascular and microvascular disease are given below.

Macrovascular disease
- Ischaemic heart disease
- Cerebrovascular disease
- Peripheral vascular disease.

Microvascular disease
- Nephropathy
- Eye: retinopathy (also cataracts)

- Neuropathy:
  - autonomic, e.g. impotence, incontinence
  - sensory, e.g. numbness, pain
  - motor, e.g. mononeuritis multiplex.

Diabetic feet

Diabetic feet illustrate the complications of diabetes very well: peripheral vascular disease predisposes the feet to ischaemic ulceration; sensory neuropathy predisposes to neuropathic ulceration. Furthermore, small vessel disease impairs wound healing, and hyperglycaemia predisposes to infection. It is therefore not surprising that gangrene and amputation of digits, feet and even legs in these patients is common.

Pathology

The two main types of diabetes have distinct pathologies.

Type I diabetes

Type I diabetes is an autoimmune disorder characterized by destruction of the beta cells of the islets of Langerhans (named after the German medical student that discovered them!) in the pancreas (which secrete insulin). It therefore results in a lack of insulin in the plasma.

Genetic factors are important, with 30–40% concordance in monozygotic (identical) twins and close linkage to HLA-DR3 and HLA-DR4.

Environmental factors are also important, and viruses such as mumps and Coxsackie viruses have been implicated as triggers for an autoimmune response directed against the beta cells.

Type II diabetes

Type II diabetes is characterized by insulin resistance, and so there are high levels of plasma insulin, but a reduced responsiveness of cells to insulin. Genetic factors are thought to be more important, as illustrated by concordance of 70–90% in monozygotic twins; however, in most cases, there seems to be a polygenic (rather than monogenic) basis for susceptibility.

Environmental factors which are important in the development of diabetes in a predisposed individual include obesity, lack of exercise and old age.

Investigations

Urinalysis for glucose

The presence of glycosuria in an individual should raise the possibility of diabetes but blood glucose measurements are needed to make the diagnosis.

Blood glucose measurement

The World Health Organization (WHO) diagnostic criteria (2000) for the diagnosis of diabetes state that a random or fasting blood glucose and, if necessary, an oral glucose tolerance test (OGTT) should be performed:

Random blood glucose

<7.0 mmol/L	diabetes excluded
>11.0 mmol/L	diabetes diagnosed
7.0–11.0 mmol/L	proceed to fasting blood glucose

Fasting blood glucose

<6.0 mmol/L	diabetes excluded
>7.0 mmol/L	diabetes diagnosed
6.0–7.0 mmol/L	proceed to OGTT

Oral glucose tolerance test

<7.8 mmol/L	diabetes excluded
>11.1 mmol/L	diabetes diagnosed
7.8–11.1 mmol/L	impaired glucose tolerance (IGT) diagnosed

Management

Diabetic management aims to control blood glucose levels, and to use other measures to reduce the complications.

Important aspects of management are patient education on diabetic diet and blood glucose monitoring to avoid hypoglycaemia and diabetic ketoacidosis.

Control of blood glucose levels

Insulin

Insulin injections must be used for type I diabetics, since they have no endogenous insulin, and is also used for type II diabetics if other treatments fail.

Most people use the human form of insulin, but a few diabetics still use bovine or porcine forms.

Insulin is administered as a subcutaneous injection. Long-, medium- and short-acting insulins are available, and are used in combination to provide glycaemic control.

A typical example of a daily insulin regime is:

- Short-acting insulin, e.g. Actrapid with each meal: 0800 h, 1200 h, 1800 h.
- Long-acting insulin, e.g. Insulatard at night: 2200 h.

Insulin has the disadvantages of having to be injected, and can cause hypoglycaemia.

Drugs

Sulphonylureas

Sulphonylureas, e.g. gliclazide, are oral hypoglycaemic drugs used for treatment of type II diabetes. They promote insulin secretion from the pancreas, but also reduce hepatic glucose release. They have the disadvantages of weight gain, and can cause hypoglycaemia.

Biguanides

Biguanides, e.g. metformin, are also used for type II diabetes. They act by promotion of insulin sensitivity. They have the advantage of promoting weight loss, but are contraindicated in renal failure, and can cause lactic acidosis.

Thiazolidinediones
Thiazolidinediones, e.g. rosiglitazone, act by promoting insulin sensitivity.

Monitoring diabetes
Glucose
Home glucose monitoring by the patient using a glucometer is done to provide guidance on the required dose of hypoglycaemic medication, e.g. insulin.

Glycosylated haemoglobin
Glycosylated haemoglobin (HbA1c) is performed to provide an estimate of glycaemic control over the previous 3 months, and is a useful measure of patient compliance with treatment. This blood test measures the proportion of red blood cells that are glycosylated. An HbA1c <8 indicates good diabetic control.

Urinalysis
Urinalysis for protein, and serum urea and electrolyte measurements, are used to detect diabetic nephropathy (renal disease).

Lipids
Serum lipids are regularly measured with the aim of reduction of hyperlipidaemia, one of the main causes of macrovascular disease.

Reduction of complications
Hypertension
Aggressive treatment of high blood pressure reduces microvascular and macrovascular complications in type II diabetes.

Hyperlipidaemia
Hyperlipidaemia should also be aggressively treated to reduce cardiovascular complications. Statins (HMG CoA reductase inhibitors) are the main drugs used.

Renal and cardiovascular complications
ACE (angiotensin-converting enzyme) inhibitors, e.g. lisinopril, have been shown to reduce the progression of renal disease and cardiovascular disease in diabetic patients. Other cardiovascular risk factors such as smoking should also be addressed.

Diabetic emergencies

Hypoglycaemia
Hypoglycaemia is the most immediately dangerous emergency and is caused by the overtreatment of diabetes with hypoglycaemic drugs, e.g. an insulin injection or the missing of a meal. Hypoglycaemia impairs cerebral function and causes autonomic stimulation, leading to sweating, hunger, irritability/anxiety, confusion, drowsiness and collapse.

Hypoglycaemia must be quickly corrected with glucose, or brain damage can result. Assess the glucose level with a BM stix. If there is any doubt about the cause, give glucose immediately as a diagnostic test. This will cause little harm in hyperglycaemic coma but will improve hypoglycaemia. *Never* give insulin, since this may cause severe brain damage or kill a hypoglycaemic patient. If the patient is conscious, immediately give glucose solution or sugar by mouth. If the patient is comatose, give sterile dextrose intravenously or glucagon intramuscularly.

Diabetic ketoacidosis

Diabetic ketoacidosis (DKA) tends to occur during periods of illness in type I diabetes, where the patient does not eat, and so does not take his insulin in the mistaken belief that he does not need it.

In DKA, very high plasma glucose levels lead to marked glycosuria and dehydration. However, the lack of insulin causes intracellular hypoglycaemia, leading to the formation of ketone bodies, thus causing acidosis.

If it is certain that collapse is due to hyperglycaemic ketoacidotic coma, the first priority is to establish an intravenous infusion line. This enables rapid rehydration to correct dehydration and electrolyte (especially potassium) losses, and the administration of insulin. Blood should be taken for baseline measurements of glucose, electrolytes, pH and blood gases. Raised plasma ketone body levels can be demonstrated with Ketostix (Ames). Medical help should be obtained as soon as possible.

Hyperosmolar non-ketotic coma

Hyperosmolar non-ketotic coma (HONC) can arise from extreme hyperglycaemia (>50 mmol/L) often caused by acute illness, and may lead to severe dehydration, which may cause renal failure and thrombosis. It is more common in type II diabetes.

Dental aspects

The main hazard is hypoglycaemia. Dental disease and treatment in particular may disrupt the normal pattern of food intake and can interfere with diabetic control and result in hypoglycaemia. It is best to give oral glucose just before the appointment and, if normal eating will be resumed at lunchtime, appointments should be early to mid-morning after a normal breakfast and normal antidiabetic treatment. Autonomic neuropathy in diabetes can cause orthostatic hypotension: supine patients should be slowly raised upright in the dental chair and helped out of it. Drugs that can disturb diabetic control – aspirin and corticosteroids – must be avoided. Any invasive treatment is best carried out in hospital.

Diabetics, even if well controlled, have a slightly more severe periodontal disease than controls. Severe dentoalveolar abscesses with fascial space involvement in seemingly healthy individuals may indicate diabetes. A dry mouth may result from dehydration and occasionally there is swelling of the salivary glands (sialosis), due to autonomic neuropathy. If control is poor, oral candidosis (candidiasis) may develop and causes, for example, angular stomatitis.

Five facts

1. Diabetes mellitus (DM) is a condition characterized by hyperglycaemia.
2. Since type I DM is caused by a complete lack of insulin, all patients need insulin.
3. Type II DM (caused by insulin resistance) may be controlled by diet, oral antihyperglycaemics or insulin.
4. Hypoglycaemia may result from the disruption of the normal pattern of food intake caused by dental disease and treatment.
5. Diabetic patients have prolonged wound healing and increased risk of infection from any dental or surgical procedure.

Epilepsy

Epilepsy is defined as the tendency to have seizures; epilepsy can therefore only be diagnosed after at least two seizures have occurred in an individual.

Since any pathology in the brain may manifest clinically with seizures, investigation for the underlying cause of seizures is essential in all individuals presenting with epilepsy.

Epidemiology

Epilepsy has an incidence of about 5/1000. Men and women are affected equally. There are two age peaks of onset of epilepsy. Most cases present in childhood or adolescence but new cases also appear in elderly people, due to their higher incidence of brain metastases.

Classification/clinical features

A seizure is any abnormal clinical event caused by abnormal electrical activity in the brain, and may be:

- generalized (loss of consciousness) or
- partial (no loss of consciousness).

Generalized seizures
Abnormal electrical activity occurs throughout the brain from the onset of the seizure. The two common types of generalized seizure are tonic–clonic (grand mal) and absence (petit mal). Other types such as myoclonic jerk, tonic and atonic also exist.

Tonic–clonic seizure (grand mal)
This is the most common form of generalized seizure. The episode may be preceded by an aura (visual symptoms). The individual then loses consciousness abruptly and becomes rigid. If standing, the individual will therefore fall to the ground. After a few seconds, the rigidity (tonic phase) is replaced by rhythmic and intermittent muscle contractions, leading to jerking movements involving the whole body (clonic phase). During this time injury may occur. Tongue biting and incontinence of urine and/or faeces may be seen. Breathing is often decreased or ceases during a seizure, which may cause cyanosis. After cessation of the seizure, the individual enters a 'post-ictal state' and can be drowsy, with a headache for an hour or so.

Absence seizure (petit mal)
Absence seizures occur mostly in childhood. The child merely becomes motionless, with a blank expression and is unresponsive to any stimuli until the episode terminates after about 10 seconds. There is no collapse. After the seizure, the child will often carry on the activity he left off (e.g. finishing the sentence he had started). Up to 30 episodes may occur in one day.

Other types of generalized seizure

Myoclonic jerk
A single muscle contraction occurs, which may for example throw the individual to the floor.

Atonic
The individual becomes flaccid, i.e. muscle tone is lost.

Tonic
A sustained period of contraction in all muscle groups occurs.

Partial seizures
Abnormal electrical activity originates from a specific localized area of the brain. Partial seizures are classified according to whether consciousness during a seizure is normal (simple partial seizure), reduced (complex partial seizure), or lost completely (secondary generalized seizure).

Simple partial seizure
Electrical activity originates from, and is confined to, a localized area of the brain; therefore, consciousness is not affected. The clinical features depend on the area of cortex exhibiting abnormal electrical activity.

Motor cortex (pre-central gyrus of frontal lobe)
Intermittent, rhythmical jerking or sustained muscle contraction may occur. A single area of the body may be affected or the attack may spread to affect other areas (*Jacksonian epilepsy*). Temporary loss of power to the affected muscle group may occur after the seizure (*Todd's paresis*).

Sensory cortex (post-central gyrus, parietal lobe)
Paraesthesia (tingling) appears and may spread to other areas.

Temporal lobe
There may be memory phenomena such as *déjà vu* (inappropriate feeling of seeing something before) or *jamais vu* (inappropriate feeling of not having seen something before). Sensory hallucinations involving smell and taste or emotional features such as fear or tearfulness may occur.

Complex partial seizure
This type of seizure results from localized electrical activity, which spreads to involve areas of the brain which control consciousness. So, although consciousness is not lost (as in a generalized seizure), it is reduced during an attack. As with a simple partial seizure, clinical features depend on the areas of the brain affected.

Secondary generalized seizure
If focal abnormal electrical activity spreads to involve the whole brain, then consciousness is lost, and the episode will resemble a generalized seizure.

Pathology

Abnormal electrical activity

The brain consists of a network of neurons (nerve cells), which are interconnected: some have an inhibitory effect on other neurons that is mediated by GABA (gamma-aminobutyric acid); others have an excitatory effect mediated by neurotransmitters such as glutamate and acetylcholine. A seizure results from an imbalance between excitatory and inhibitory activity. Cyclical bursts of abnormal neuronal activity therefore occur, associated with the seizure. In fact, imbalances of neurotransmitter levels are implicated in many psychiatric conditions such as depression and schizophrenia.

Pathological causes of epilepsy

Any pathology of the brain parenchyma (substance) may cause a seizure. A classification of causes is listed below:

- *Idiopathic* (unknown): this is by far the majority of cases of child or adolescent-onset epilepsy.
- *Infarction*: stroke damages a focal area of brain, so tends to cause partial seizures.
- *Neoplasia*: cerebral neoplasms are usually secondary (e.g. carcinoma of breast, lung, gastrointestinal, melanoma) but primary tumours include glioma, meningioma and ependymoma.
- *Structural abnormalities*: arteriovenous malformations (such as in von-Hippel–Lindau syndrome, Sturge–Weber syndrome and neurofibromatosis type II) and hydrocephalus may interrupt the normal architecture of the brain parenchyma. Trauma also leads to interruption of the normal architecture of the parenchyma.
- *Infection*: meningitis (infection of the meninges and cerebrospinal fluid) or encephalitis (infection of the brain parenchyma) tend to cause generalized or secondary generalized seizures.

  Encephalitis is principally caused by viruses such as herpes simplex virus (HSV), Japanese B encephalitis (a flavivirus) and HIV. In Europe, most cases are caused by HSV. It most commonly infects the temporal lobes, and can lead to complex partial seizures with temporal lobe features (see above).

  Localized infection such as cerebral abscess, toxoplasmosis and cysticercosis may act on a focal part of the brain to cause partial seizures.
- *Inflammation*: vasculitis (e.g. systemic lupus erythematosus (SLE)) leads to small vessel ischaemia and associated neuronal death, and may therefore cause generalized seizures, as well as neuropsychiatric disturbances.
- *Metabolic disturbances* may lead to generalized seizures. Examples are:
  - hypoglycaemia, e.g. diabetes mellitus, alcoholism, malnutrition
  - hypo/hypernatraemia
  - hypocalcaemia, e.g. hypoparathyroidism, osteomalacia
  - hypomagnesaemia
  - liver failure.
- *Drug* examples are:
  - alcohol and other drugs of abuse
  - psychotropics – phenothiazines, tricyclic antidepressants
  - antibiotics – penicillin, isoniazid
  - antimalarials – chloroquine, mefloquine.

- *Degenerative brain diseases* such as Alzheimer's disease, Pick's disease and Creutzfeldt–Jakob disease (CJD) may all promote seizures.

Investigations

An electroencephalogram (EEG) measures the pattern of electrical activity in the brain and is used to establish the diagnosis and characterize the type of epilepsy. If characteristic changes are seen (sharp waves or spikes), then this is highly specific for epilepsy.

Imaging of the brain with magnetic resonance imaging (MRI) or computed tomography (CT) should be done to detect any structural cause for seizures such as neoplasm, trauma, infarction, abscess or AV (arteriovenous) malformation.

It is absolutely vital to measure serum metabolites, since they account for the majority of cases of hospital seizures in patients with no known epilepsy. Thus, serum glucose, liver function tests, urea and electrolytes (including sodium), calcium and magnesium should always be measured.

Cerebrospinal fluid (CSF) needs to be examined in order to look for infective causes of seizures. However, a lumbar puncture should only be performed after a CT or MRI of the brain has excluded a mass lesion (otherwise this could cause fatal herniation of the brain through the foramen magnum if CSF is removed from the spine). The CSF obtained is sent for microscopy to detect bacteria (Gram stain), cryptococcus (Indian ink stain), TB (auramine stain) or malignant cells (e.g. lymphoma). Polymerase chain reaction (PCR) analysis may be performed to detect HSV.

An HIV test should be performed if features suggesting immunosuppression are seen. This includes the diagnosis of cryptococcosis, TB or lymphomatous meningitis. (See chapter on HIV and AIDS.)

Management

Anticonvulsant drugs
Drug treatment is normally initiated once an individual has had more than one seizure. The choice of drug depends mainly on the type of epilepsy. Table 1 provides a summary of first-line (used first) and second-line (used if first-line drug fails) drug therapy for epilepsy, together with common side effects. Note that all of the main anticonvulsants except gabapentin are uncommonly associated with rashes and bone marrow dysfunction. Some drugs such as phenytoin and carbamazepine require periodic drug level monitoring to ensure their efficacy.

Epilepsy is well-controlled in the majority of individuals on a single anticonvulsant; however, adverse effects can be troublesome (see Table 1). Therefore, after control of seizures for at least 2 years, it may be decided to discontinue anticonvulsant medication; about 60% of people remain seizure-free, but the rest have to recommence medication.

Driving regulations
For normal drivers, driving is not permitted within 1 year of a single, first seizure. In established epilepsy, driving is not permitted within 1 year of the most recent seizure. An exception to this rule is where seizures have occurred only at night for the last

Table 1 First-line and second-line anticonvulsant drugs together with important side effects for the major types of epilepsy

Type of epilepsy	First line (drug which is tried first)	Second line
Generalized (tonic–clonic)	Sodium valproate (drowsiness, cerebellar signs)	Lamotrigine (drowsiness, ataxia) Carbamazepine (drowsiness, cerebellar signs, SIADH[1])
Generalized (absence)	Ethosuximide (dizziness, ataxia)	Sodium valproate
Partial	Carbamazepine	Lamotrigine Sodium valproate Gabapentin (drowsiness, ataxia) Phenytoin (drowsiness, cerebellar signs, liver dysfunction, gingival swelling)

[1]SIADH, syndrome of inappropriate antidiuretic hormone.

3 years. Driving is also not permitted during and within 6 months of withdrawal of anticonvulsant medication. Heavy goods vehicle (HGV) drivers are not permitted to drive unless free of medication and seizures for 10 years.

Basic management of a seizure
An epileptic seizure is a medical emergency.

1. The principles of basic life support (BLS) should be employed: check airway, breathing and circulation (ABC). Note: do not put your finger inside the mouth of a person during a seizure, since involuntary closure of the mouth may occur.
2. Prevent injury to the patient. Move the patient away from any hazard such as furniture or dental equipment. The head should be held and supported in order to prevent it hitting the ground during the seizure.
3. Most seizures terminate spontaneously. If the seizure has not terminated within 5 min, urgent medical attention should be sought.
4. After a seizure, the patient will be post-ictal, and therefore unconscious. Re-check ABC, and then put the patient in the recovery position in order to prevent aspiration.

Status epilepticus
If a seizure persists beyond 30 min or is recurrent (without recovery in between seizures), the patient is in *status epilepticus*. Medical attention should be sought immediately, but management consists of:

- high-flow oxygen via a face mask
- intravenous (IV) access and 10 mg IV rectal diazepam
- BM stix for blood glucose measurement

- urgent serum biochemistry for assay of glucose, sodium, liver function test (LFT), calcium and magnesium, and immediate correction if abnormal
- further diazepam after 15 min if seizures persist
- oxygenation monitored with arterial blood gases
- IV phenytoin may terminate seizure (but must be given with cardiac monitoring because of risk of tachyarrhythmias)
- intubation with ventilation and emergency transfer to intensive care unit if seizures persist beyond 30 min, or if, despite oxygen therapy, hypoxia is present.

Pseudoseizure

One cause of apparent seizure activity not responsive to treatment is *pseudoseizure*. Although seizure-like behaviour (waving of arms, jerking) occurs, the EEG is normal, i.e. there is no actual epileptic activity! This psychiatric condition can be extremely difficult to diagnose. Therefore, when faced with someone fitting, you *must* assume that it is genuine and treat the individual appropriately. In other words, do *not* try to diagnose a pseudoseizure yourself!

Dental aspects

In the past, particularly, gingival swelling due to phenytoin required treatment by gingival surgery.

Convulsions may have craniofacial sequelae, especially lacerations, haematomas and fractures. Trauma frequently results from a grand mal attack when the patient falls unconscious or from the muscle spasm. Such injuries can include:

- fractures of the vertebrae or limbs
- dislocations
- periorbital subcutaneous haematomas in the absence of facial fractures
- injuries to the face from falling (lacerations, haematomas, fractures of the facial skeleton)
- fractures, devitalization, subluxation or loss of teeth (a chest radiograph may be required)
- subluxation of the temporomandibular joint (TMJ)
- lacerations or scarring of tongue, lips or buccal mucosa.

Epileptics can have good and bad phases and dental treatment should be carried out in a good phase, when attacks are infrequent. Individuals who have infrequent seizures, or who depend on others (such as those with a learning impairment), may fail to take regular medication and thus be poorly controlled. When carrying out dental treatment in a known epileptic, a strong mouth prop should be kept in position and the oral cavity kept as free as possible of debris. As much apparatus as possible should be kept away from the area around the patient.

Drugs, e.g. metronidazole, can be epileptogenic or interfere with anticonvulsants, or their own effects can be altered by anticonvulsant therapy and they are therefore contraindicated.

Five facts

1. A seizure is any abnormal clinical event caused by abnormal electrical activity in the brain.
2. Epilepsy is the tendency to have seizures (i.e. at least two seizures).
3. Diazepam (IV or per rectal) is the best way to acutely terminate a seizure.
4. Seizures may be generalized (loss of consciousness) or partial (no loss of consciousness).
5. When carrying out dental treatment in a known epileptic, a strong mouth prop should be kept in position and the oral cavity kept as free as possible from debris.

Gallstones

Risk factors

Gallstones are common, occurring in >20% of middle-aged women. There are five classic risk factors for gallstones (the 5 F's):

- Female
- Fair
- Fat
- Fertile
- Forty.

Other predisposing factors include:

- excess mucus production by the gall bladder
- biliary infection
- biliary stasis (e.g. in pregnancy)
- ileal dysfunction (prevents reabsorption of bile)
- obesity
- hypercholesterolaemia
- chronic liver disease.

Physiology

Bile is composed of cholesterol, phospholipids, bile salts, water and conjugated bilirubin, the breakdown product of haemoglobin. Cholesterol is hydrophobic (i.e. not water soluble) and is therefore transported in bile along with bile salts and phospholipids in water-soluble micelles. In the bowel, the bile salts break down and emulsify the cholesterol to facilitate its absorption. The bile salts then get absorbed into the portal circulation and are taken to the liver, for further secretion in the bile. This enterohepatic circulation allows a small amount of bile salts to circulate up to 10 times a day.

There are three types of gallstones:

- mixed (75%)
- cholesterol (20%)
- pigment (5%).

Cholesterol stones result from supersaturation of bile with cholesterol, more commonly due to a deficiency of bile salts – as occurs after resection of the terminal ileum – than from hypercholesterolaemia. Pigment stones are small and black; they are composed of calcium bilirubinate with or without calcium carbonate. These form due to excess bile pigment being deposited in the biliary tract, and are therefore often the result of haemolytic anaemias (e.g. sickle cell disease).

Pathology

Most gallstones are symptomless but some can result in a remarkable range of problems.

Silent
The majority of gallstones are *asymptomatic* and are discovered incidentally, e.g. from an abdominal X-ray taken for other reasons. Here, the gallstones lie free in the lumen of the gall bladder and cause no pathological disturbance.

Obstruction of the cystic duct
- When a gallstone becomes impacted in the gall bladder at its exit (Hartmann's pouch) or in the cystic duct, then obstruction will occur. Water is absorbed from the bile in the gall bladder, and the bile then becomes concentrated, resulting in a chemical cholecystitis. Although initially this is sterile, it becomes secondarily infected with bacteria to produce *acute cholecystitis*.
- Repeated attacks of the above can lead to chronic fibrosis and thickening of the gall bladder wall, causing *chronic cholecystitis*.
- Sometimes the obstructed gall bladder is empty, and then the gall bladder can become distended and secrete excess mucus, leading to a *mucocele*.

Gallstone in the common bile duct
This condition may be asymptomatic or distend the common bile duct (CBD) proximal to the obstruction, causing colicky pain – *biliary colic*. If there is complete obstruction of the CBD, *obstructive jaundice* can result. If combined with infection, the patient can become systemically unwell, with pyrexia, jaundice and pain (Charcot's triad) – *cholangitis*.

Gallstone ulcerating through the gall bladder
Here the stone can migrate into the neighbouring bowel, typically the duodenum. The stone can then travel down the bowel and impact in the distal ileum, resulting in small bowel obstruction – *gallstone ileus*.

Chronic irritation and/or carcinogenic effects of bile
The presence of gallstones for a number of years may cause a chronic irritation to the gall bladder. This condition, combined with the potential carcinogenic effect of some of the bile constituents, can predispose to *carcinoma of the gall bladder*.

Gallstone obstructing pancreatic drainage
- Gallstones in the CBD distal to the entry of the main pancreatic duct of Wirsung (i.e. below the level of the sphincter of Oddi) can cause obstruction of pancreatic drainage, leading to *acute pancreatitis*.
- Repeated attacks of the above can lead to a gradual destruction of the functioning pancreatic tissue – *chronic pancreatitis*.

Clinical syndromes

Biliary colic
- The impaction of the gallstone within Hartmann's pouch or the cystic duct causes the proximal biliary tree to periodically contract in an attempt to relieve the obstruction. This results in an intermittent pain (colic).

- In biliary colic the pain is usually in the right upper quadrant (RUQ) or epigastrium and may radiate to the tip of the right shoulder; it is often accompanied by waves of nausea and vomiting.
- Management involves pain relief, often using antispasmodics such as Buscopan (hyoscine).

Acute cholecystitis
- Systemic signs of infection include:
  - fever
  - raised white blood cell (WBC) count
  - malaise
  - anorexia.
- RUQ tenderness and/or mass (distended, inflamed gall bladder wrapped in the 'abdominal policeman' of the omentum).
- Complications include:
  - empyema (pus-filled gall bladder)
  - obstructive jaundice (if the inflamed gall bladder presses on the CBD).
- Management includes pain relief, antibiotics and resting the gastrointestinal tract (i.e. keep nil by mouth). This is followed by cholecystectomy (usually laparoscopic), usually around 6 weeks later.

Chronic cholecystitis
- This condition classically presents with recurrent bouts of biliary colic (recurrent mild acute attacks), typically after eating fatty foods, as the fat in the diet provokes release of cholecystokinin, which causes gall bladder contraction.
- Management is by elective cholecystectomy.

Obstructive jaundice
- Obstructive jaundice is associated with icterus (jaundice), pruritus (itching), dark urine and pale stools (as the bile pigment is excreted in the urine instead of the stools).
- Management involves identifying the cause: if gallstones are found in the CBD, this is usually dealt with by ERCP (endoscopic retrograde cholangiopancreatography; see below), with or without sphincterotomy; if the cause is carcinoma of the head of the pancreas, then the options are usually palliative surgical bypass, surgical resection (Whipple's procedure) or symptom-directed conservative management.

Ascending cholangitis
- Here, the CBD is distended and filled with pus, leading to a life-threatening septicaemia.
- Immediate surgical drainage is required.

Courvoisier's law

Ludwig Courvoisier, the famous Swiss professor of surgery, stated:

'If in the presence of jaundice the gall bladder is palpable, then the cause is not likely to be gallstones.'

This is because if the obstruction causing the jaundice was due to gallstones, the gall bladder would be thickened and fibrotic, and thus cannot distend. However, obstruction of the gall bladder from other causes, most importantly carcinoma of the head of pancreas, is associated with a normal gall bladder, which can therefore dilate.

Investigations

- Liver function tests: may suggest obstructive jaundice (raised serum bilirubin and alkaline phosphatase).
- Plain abdominal X-ray: shows gallstones in 10% of cases.
- Abdominal ultrasound: the mainstay of investigation, and can show gallstones, gall bladder wall thickness and, very importantly, the diameter of the CBD (and thus whether it is dilated or not).
- Computed tomography (CT), cholecystograms, cholangiography and HIDA (hepatobiliary iminodiacetic acid) scanning: these specialist investigations are only used in certain situations.
- ERCP: a technique of endoscopic intubation of the bile ducts through the ampulla of Vater. Radio-opaque dye is then injected to give images of the biliary tract. Calculi may be removed using a Dormia basket, often after first dividing the sphincter of Oddi (sphincterotomy).

Cholecystectomy

Cholecystectomy is the main treatment for most gallstone disease and has superseded medical management of stone dissolution. Laparoscopic cholecystectomy was the first common 'keyhole' surgical procedure performed, and has become so popular that open operation is virtually never performed as first-line treatment. Most patients can be discharged from hospital within 48 hours and return to work by 2 weeks postoperatively. However, like all operations, cholecystectomy can cause complications (chest infection, thromboembolic disease, bleeding, etc.); specific complications can include:

- biliary peritonitis (from a bile leak due to damage to the biliary tract intraoperatively)
- jaundice (due to inadvertent ligature of the CBD or damage to the pancreas or its drainage).

Five facts

1. Gallstones occur in >20% of middle-aged women.
2. Gallstones can present with pain, jaundice, infection, pancreatitis and possibly even malignancy.
3. Ultrasound is the first-line investigation of choice.
4. Ascending cholangitis is a surgical emergency, characterized by fever, pain and jaundice (Charcot's triad).
5. Laparoscopic cholecystectomy is a common 'keyhole' surgical procedure with good results.

Gastrointestinal bleeding

Gastrointestinal haemorrhage may be from the upper gastrointestinal (UGI) or the lower gastrointestinal (LGI) tract, the demarcation being at the ligament of Treitz (a fibromuscular band that suspends the distal duodenum at the duodenojejunal junction). UGI bleeding presents with haematemesis and melaena, whereas LGI bleeding presents with frank, red blood PR (per rectum).

Management principles are to:

- assess and replace the blood loss (see chapter on shock and haemorrhage)
- diagnose the cause
- treat and control the cause of the bleeding.

Causes

Bleeding may be because of general causes of bleeding (see chapter on bleeding tendency) or may be specific to the GI tract (as shown in Table 1).

Table 1 Causes of upper gastrointestinal (UGI) and lower gastrointestinal (LGI) bleeding

UGI bleeding	LGI bleeding
Peptic oesophagitis	Colorectal adenoma and carcinoma
Oesophageal varices	Diverticular disease
Peptic ulcer	Angiodysplasia
Gastric erosions	Inflammatory bowel disease
Mallory–Weiss tears (from vomiting)	Haemorrhoids (piles)
Stomach cancer	
Meckel's diverticulitis	

Upper gastrointestinal bleeding

Peptic ulcer disease (PUD) and erosions due to chronic use of non-steroidal anti-inflammatory drugs (NSAIDs) and/or steroids account for the vast majority of UGI bleeds in the UK. Oesophageal varices, which are dilated, tortuous veins at the lower end of the oesophagus due to portal hypertension from cirrhosis, account for roughly 10% of cases of UGI haemorrhage. Mallory–Weiss tears are mucosal tears of the upper part of the stomach due to repeated vomits, typically after an alcoholic binge. A Meckel's diverticulum is an embryological remnant of the vitello-intestinal duct that is present in 2% of the general population, which, if it gets inflamed, can bleed.

Oesophagogastroduodenoscopy is the mainstay of diagnosis. Varices may be compressed with a Sengstaken–Blakemore balloon. Bleeding PUs are usually treated with an intravenous proton pump inhibitor (PPI) infusion and/or endoscopic diathermy or an injection of adrenaline (epinephrine) into the ulcer base. If medical management fails, open surgical exploration may be required in order to ligate the offending blood vessel.

Lower gastrointestinal bleeding

Colonoscopy, angiography or a white cell scan may be used to locate the source of bleeding.

Angiodysplasia
Angiodysplasia is a condition of mucosal or submucosal vascular malformations, most often in the caecum or ascending colon. Colonoscopic diathermy or resection may be required.

Diverticular disease
Diverticular disease (DD) is a condition whereby the mucosa of the bowel (typically the sigmoid colon, descending colon and caecum) herniates through the muscle wall to give rise to multiple outpouchings termed diverticula. These are thought to arise from a chronic increase in intraluminal pressure causing the herniations, and are thus commoner with increasing age. Diets that are low in fibre do not distend the colon and have a tendency to cause constipation, thereby increasing the intraluminal pressure and predisposing to DD, which might explain why DD is far more common in Western countries.

If a diverticulum becomes infected, the condition is called diverticulitis. Acute diverticulitis is managed with antibiotics (typically cefuroxime plus metronidazole) and 'drip and suck' (intravenous fluids and nasogastric aspiration). Inflamed diverticula can either perforate, causing peritonitis, pericolic abscess or colovesical fistula, or bleed, causing LGI haemorrhage. DD is the commonest cause of sudden, profuse, bright red PR bleeding in an elderly patient and often requires surgical management.

Haemorrhoids
Haemorrhoids are dilated rectal veins typically found at the 3, 7 and 11 o'clock positions around the anus. They may be classified as follows:

- 1st degree - the piles bleed but do not prolapse
- 2nd degree - the piles prolapse on defaecation but reduce spontaneously
- 3rd degree - the piles prolapse on defaecation and require manual reduction by the patient's finger
- 4th degree - the piles remain persistently prolapsed outside the anal verge.

Bleeding from haemorrhoids ('piles') is rarely torrential and is unlikely to need surgical management in the acute setting. Piles can usually be managed conservatively with avoidance of straining at defaecation, laxatives and glyceryl trinitrate (GTN) ointment. They may also be sclerosed with 5% phenol injected above each pile, or may be banded, resulting in strangulation of the pile. Haemorrhoidectomy tends to be reserved for 3rd- and 4th-degree piles.

Five facts

1. GI haemorrhage may be due to general bleeding diatheses or causes specific to the GI tract.
2. UGI haemorrhage is most often due to peptic ulcer disease.
3. Intravenous PPIs are an important part of the management of UGI bleeding from peptic ulcers.
4. Diverticular disease is the commonest cause of severe LGI haemorrhage in the elderly.
5. Haemorrhoids do not usually cause significant PR bleeding and can be managed by GTN ointment, banding, sclerotherapy or surgery.

Haematological malignancies

Haematological malignancies are a range of disorders characterized by malignant proliferation of blood cells. Most affect the white blood cells (WBCs): either lymphoid cells (e.g. lymphocytes) or myeloid cells (e.g. neutrophils). If this process occurs in the bone marrow, it is called leukaemia; if it occurs in the reticuloendothelial system (lymphatics, lymph nodes and spleen), it is termed lymphoma.

These malignant diseases (lymphoreticular malignancies) are potentially lethal and, since lymphoid tissue is spread throughout the body, they have wide-ranging effects.

Leukaemia

The aetiology of leukaemias includes:

- genetic predisposition (e.g. in patients with Down syndrome)
- ionizing radiation (leukaemia was common after the Chernobyl nuclear accident)
- chemicals (e.g. benzene)
- viruses.

Leukaemias are classified by:

- clinical course (acute or chronic)
- cell of origin (lymphoblast or non-lymphoblast).

Acute leukaemias

Acute leukaemias are malignant neoplasms of immature WBCs in the bone marrow and are characterized by primitive blast cells in the blood and bone marrow. They account for nearly 50% of all malignant disease in children. They follow an acute and aggressive course.

There are two main types of acute leukaemia:

- acute lymphoblastic leukaemia (ALL) – proliferation of lymphoblasts
- acute myeloid leukaemia (AML) – proliferation of myeloid precursors.

Clinical features
Both AML and ALL have similar features:

- non-tender generalized lymphadenopathy and splenomegaly
- pallor due to anaemia
- bruising due to thrombocytopenia.

Immunosuppression is either due to leukaemia itself or neutropenia associated with chemotherapy. Organisms that are particularly important in neutropenia are:

- Gram-positive bacteria: *Staphylococcus*.
- Gram-negative bacteria: *Escherichia coli, Klebsiella, Pseudomonas*.
- Fungi: *Candida, Pneumocystis carinii*.
- Viruses: herpes viruses, e.g. herpes simplex virus, varicella zoster virus and cytomegalovirus (CMV).

Pathology
Acute leukaemia rapidly infiltrates the bone marrow, therefore crowding out other cells and leading to anaemia and thrombocytopenia.

Leukaemia cells eventually 'spill over' into the bloodstream. Cells may infiltrate other tissues. Note that ALL has a propensity for spread to the central nervous system.

Investigations
Bone marrow and blood film
Blast cells are the dominant type. Numbers of erythrocytes, mature leukocytes and platelets may be heavily diminished, which indicates bone marrow failure. Blast cells are larger than mature cells and they have large nuclei. In AML, there is an Auer rod seen in the cytoplasm of the blast cell, which distinguishes it from ALL.

Immunological, genetic and chromosomal markers
These markers may be used to distinguish AML from ALL, and between their various subtypes.

The above investigations are supplemented by chest radiography, computed tomography (CT) and magnetic resonance imaging (MRI) scans and by lumbar puncture.

Chronic leukaemias
Chronic leukaemias are malignant proliferations of mature WBCs characterized by an excess of mature leukocytes in blood and bone marrow and are mainly diseases of adult life. They are chronic disorders but may progress to acute leukaemia.

Chronic leukaemias may be divided into:

- chronic lymphocytic leukaemia (CLL) – proliferation of mature lymphocytes
- chronic myeloid leukaemia (CML) – proliferation of mature myeloid cells, e.g. neutrophils, basophils, eosinophils.

Clinical features
The constitutional symptoms of fever, tiredness and weight loss are common to both types of chronic leukaemia. Patients with CML are most commonly between 40 and 70 years old. They may present with splenomegaly, which is massive in a minority of cases. Hepatomegaly may also occur, but lymphadenopathy is uncommon. CLL tends to occur in the elderly. Patients may present with painless lymphadenopathy or splenomegaly. Chronic leukaemias are less aggressive than acute leukaemias, so are less likely to cause bruising (low platelets) and marked anaemia.

Pathology
CML is an expansion of granulocytes, including neutrophils, basophils and eosinophils. Ninety per cent of cases of CML are associated with the Philadelphia chromosome mutation. This is a translocation between chromosomes 9 and 22. The *bcr* gene on chromosome 22 fuses with the *abl* gene on chromosome 9, thereby creating a gene with oncogenic (cancer-causing) activity.

Acute transformation
After a variable period of time, CML undergoes transformation into the more aggressive AML. This AML tends to be resistant to treatment, and has a high mortality.

CLL is due to a monoclonal expansion of B lymphocytes. These B cells do not differentiate to produce antibodies; therefore, patients are immunocompromised. CLL generally does not undergo acute transformation.

Investigations

Blood film and bone marrow
Increased numbers of the mature clonal cells may be seen. The cells are morphologically identical to normal cells. There may be depression of erythrocyte and platelet numbers.

Immunological, genetic and chromosomal markers
These markers include the Philadelphia chromosome (see above).

The above investigations are supplemented by chest radiography, CT and MRI scans.

Treatment of leukaemias

Chemotherapy
Cytotoxic drugs are used to kill the rapidly proliferating cells. They therefore preferentially affect malignant cells, although other cells may be affected, e.g. hair follicles. Bone marrow suppression is a common side effect, which may lead to neutropenia, and therefore predisposition to infection and sepsis.

Combinations of 3–4 drugs are used to treat leukaemia. Some of the common drugs used are listed in Table 1. (Note that the combination of agents used for each malignancy is outside the syllabus of dental undergraduate exams.) The mechanisms and side effects of cytotoxic agents are given in Table 2.

Table 1 Common chemotherapy agents used to treat leukaemia

Malignant disease	Disease subgroup	Agents
Acute leukaemias	ALL	Vincristine, prednisolone, asparaginase, daunorubicin
	AML	Daunorubicin and cytosine arabinoside
Chronic leukaemias	CLL	Sometimes chlorambucil
	CML	Hydroxycarbamide
Lymphomas	Hodgkin's disease	ABVD or MOPP
	Non-Hodgkin's lymphomas	CHOP

ABVD = Adriamycin, bleomycin, vinblastine, dacarbazine.
MOPP = mustine (chlormethine), Oncovin (vincristine), procarbazine, prednisolone.
CHOP = cyclophosphamide, doxorubicin hydrochloride, Oncovin, prednisolone.

Table 2 Mechanisms and side effects of cytotoxic agents

Cytotoxic agent	Mechanism	Characteristic side effect
Antimetabolites, e.g. methotrexate, 6-mercaptopurine	Inhibit nucleotide incorporation into DNA during its synthesis	Gastrointestinal toxicity
DNA-binding agents, e.g. daunorubicin, adriamycin	Inhibit DNA replication	Cardiac toxicity
Vinca alkaloids, e.g. vincristine, vinblastine	Inhibit DNA replication	Peripheral neuropathy
Alkylating agents, e.g. cyclophosphamide	Cross-linking of DNA	Haemorrhagic cystitis (inflammation of the bladder)

Prophylactic antibiotics/antifungal agents are given to reduce the incidence of neutropenic sepsis and fungal infection.

Transfusion for anaemia and thrombocytopenia
Transfusion of red blood cells or platelets should be given for anaemia and thrombocytopenia, respectively.

Dental aspects
Oropharyngeal lesions, which can be the presenting complaint in leukaemia, include bleeding and petechiae, mucosal pallor and sometimes gingival swelling, oral ulceration, pericoronitis and cervical lymphadenopathy. Herpetic oral and perioral infection is common and troublesome, as are varicella zoster infections. Candidiasis is particularly common in the oral cavity and the paranasal sinuses, and aspergillosis or mucormycosis can involve the maxillary antrum and be invasive.

Myeloma

Myeloma is a malignant proliferation of plasma cells. Plasma cells are B cells that have differentiated to produce antibodies. Myeloma cells produce paraprotein, which consists of a monoclonal proliferation of either whole antibodies, or light chain precursors of antibodies. If the paraprotein is a light chain, it may appear in the urine, where it is referred to as Bence–Jones protein. Plasma cell diseases are sometimes termed monoclonal gammopathies, or paraproteinaemias. The malignant plasma cells produce defective immunoglobulins and release osteoclast-activating factors, which cause bone resorption and pain.

Myeloma thus produces a range of clinical features:

- bone marrow suppression due to infiltration
- lytic lesions in the bones due to cytokine stimulation of osteoclastic bone resorption, e.g. pepper pot appearance on skull X-ray
- renal failure, mainly due to light chain filtration by the kidneys
- infection, due to hypogammaglobulinaemia (deficiency of antibodies)
- amyloidosis may arise.

Investigations
Blood film and bone marrow
Myeloma cells are seen.

Serum protein electrophoresis
This reveals the paraprotein.

Urine protein electrophoresis
This will reveal the Bence–Jones protein if present.

Serum calcium
Serum calcium is raised due to bone resorption.

Skeletal radiographic survey or bone scan
Lytic bone lesions may be seen.

Treatment
Symptomatic patients, or those with progressive bone lesions or worsening paraproteinaemia, are treated with chemotherapy.

New treatments include interferon, thalidomide, bone marrow transplantation and haematopoietic growth factors. The prognosis is poor, with a 3-year mean survival.

Transfusion is used for anaemia and thrombocytopenia.

Dental aspects
The skull, especially the calvarium, is ultimately affected with rounded, discrete (punched-out) osteolytic lesions in about 70% of cases. Jaw lesions are seen less frequently.

Lymphomas

Lymphomas are malignant proliferations of lymphocytes in the reticuloendothelial system. There are two types:

- Hodgkin's lymphoma (also known as Hodgkin's disease), named after Thomas Hodgkin of Guy's Hospital, London.
- Non-Hodgkins lymphoma:
  - high grade
  - low grade.

Most lymphomas are non-Hodgkin's lymphomas (NHL).

Hodgkin's lymphoma
Hodgkin's lymphoma is characterized by the presence of the Reed–Sternberg cell, which is derived from B cells. Reed–Sternberg cells are surrounded by a host of T cells, eosinophils and other cells.

There are four main types of Hodgkin's lymphoma:

- lymphocyte-predominant (best prognosis)
- nodular sclerosing

- mixed cellularity
- lymphocyte-depleted (worst prognosis).

Adults from the age of 30 to 60 years old are most commonly affected.

Clinical features
- *B-symptoms*: an unexplained fever >38°C, night sweats and loss of >10% body weight are each referred to as B-symptoms. The presence of B-symptoms suggests more aggressive disease. The fever may cycle with periods of normal temperature, in which case it is called a Pel–Ebstein fever.
- *Pruritus* may occur, and may be severe.
- *Alcohol-induced pain* is also a characteristic feature of Hodgkin's lymphoma.
- *Painless, rubbery lymphadenopathy* is a common presenting feature. Mediastinal lymphadenopathy may cause superior vena cava (SVC) obstruction (see chapter on lung cancer) or bronchial obstruction/collapse. Oropharyngeal lymphadenopathy may cause a sore throat or stridor/airway obstruction. Characteristically, contiguous spread of Hodgkin's disease occurs (in contrast to non-Hodgkin's lymphoma).
- *Hepatosplenomegaly* may also occur.

Non-Hodgkin's lymphoma
Non-Hodgkin's lymphoma is best thought of as the reticuloendothelial equivalent to lymphocytic leukaemia. NHL may be either high grade (equivalent to acute leukaemia) or low grade (equivalent to chronic lymphoma). Furthermore, NHL may be either B cell (most common) or T cell in origin.

The average age of presentation with lymphoma is 50 years, but high grade lymphomas often present in young adults.

Clinical features
- *Painless lymphadenopathy* is the most common presenting complaint.
- *Constitutional symptoms* of night sweats, pruritus and weight loss are less common than in Hodgkin's disease.
- *Hepatosplenomegaly* may occur.
- *Bone marrow involvement* in aggressive disease causes bone marrow suppression to occur.
- *Involvement of other organs*, e.g. brain, testis, thyroid, spinal cord and gastrointestinal tract.

Pathology
Most cases are idiopathic. However, some conditions may predispose to lymphoma:

- immunosuppressed individuals and patients with AIDS are predisposed to lymphoma, which may be associated with Epstein–Barr virus infection.
- autoimmune diseases such as coeliac disease and pernicious anaemia predispose to gastrointestinal lymphoma.

Investigations for lymphoma

Full blood count and blood film
In advanced disease, bone marrow suppression may occur. Lymphoma cells are uncommonly found in the peripheral blood film.

Lymph node biopsy
A lymph node biopsy is required to establish the diagnosis of lymphoma. Immunohistochemistry, genetic and chromosomal markers may be used to distinguish subtypes of lymphoma.

Computed tomography
A CT scan is needed to assess the extent of spread of disease, and therefore stage it.

Treatment of lymphomas
Treatment often includes chemotherapy, given in various combination regimes, and irradiation:

- Radiotherapy is used to treat localized disease without distal spread. It is also used to shrink down lymphadenopathy, causing compression of surrounding tissue, e.g. SVC obstruction.
- Chemotherapy – see treatment of leukaemia.
- Transfusion for anaemia and thrombocytopenia if required.

Dental aspects
Painless enlarged cervical lymph nodes are the initial complaint in 50% of lymphomas, but oral lesions are uncommon. Oral infections, especially with viruses and fungi, may be seen. NHL may occur in the mouth in AIDS.

Five facts

1. Leukaemia is the malignant proliferation of white blood cells in the bone marrow.
2. Lymphoma is the malignant proliferation of lymphocytes in the reticuloendothelial system (lymphatics, lymph nodes and spleen).
3. Lymphoma is histologically classified as either Hodgkin's or non-Hodgkin's.
4. Oropharyngeal lesions in leukaemia include bleeding and petechiae, mucosal pallor, gingival swelling, oral ulceration, pericoronitis and cervical lymphadenopathy.
5. All haematological malignancies cause immunosuppression, which predisposes to oral infections such as herpes simplex, varicella zoster infections and candidiasis.

Head injury

Every year, over one million patients present to Accident & Emergency departments in the UK with head injuries. Around 10% of these are admitted, and over 3000 patients are transferred to neurosurgical centres every year. 60% of head injury patients are adults, of which 70% are male, and 25% have a preceding history of alcohol intake.

Assaults and road traffic accidents are the major causes, with alcohol or other drugs being a frequent cofactor. Violence (assaults or fights) is increasingly common but since the institution of seat-belt wearing, head injury from road accidents is not. Industrial accidents, sport and epilepsy are other causes. Most head injuries are in previously fit young men, because of their risk behaviour. Children, particularly before they have perfected their walking skills, are also uniquely susceptible to head trauma because of their risk behaviour and higher cranial mass to body mass ratio.

Classification

Head injuries can be classified by:

- severity (mild, moderate or severe)
- mechanism (blunt vs penetrating)
- morphology (skull fracture vs intracranial injury).

Intracranial injuries can be:

- focal (extradural, subdural or intracerebral)
- diffuse (concussion or diffuse axonal injury).

Early complications

Death may result immediately from brain damage, airway obstruction or damage to other vital organs such as the heart. Of survivors with brain damage, 12% die within 2 days. The brain can be fatally damaged without fracture of the skull or even a blemish on the scalp.

Conscious level

Many patients are brought into the emergency department confused, concussed or in a coma. The brain is invariably damaged in those who have lost consciousness, and sometimes in those who have not, and many are suffering effects from alcohol or other drugs of misuse. Concussion, an immediate but transient loss of consciousness, is always associated with a short period of amnesia, and there is some brain damage even if after-effects are not detectable on neurological testing, cerebrospinal fluid (CSF) examination, computed tomography (CT) or magnetic resonance imaging (MRI). With diffuse brain damage, there is usually amnesia both for the traumatic event, and afterwards (post-traumatic amnesia) for a period far exceeding that of unconsciousness.

Consciousness may not necessarily be lost if brain damage is local, e.g. when the skull is penetrated by a sharp object. Maintenance of consciousness does not therefore imply the absence of brain damage; 30% of patients with ultimately fatal head injuries may talk after injury and some are completely lucid for a time. Prolonged unconsciousness, when there are no complications such as haematomas and where there are no focal signs, is caused by severe brain damage or other unrelated disease.

Glasgow Coma Scale
First described in Glasgow, UK, the Glasgow Coma Scale (GCS) is a widely used scoring system to assess consciousness. It is divided into three components: eyes (E), motor response (M) and verbal response (V).

Eyes (E)
1. No opening
2. Eyes open to pain
3. Eyes open to verbal command
4. Eyes open spontaneously

Motor (M)
1. No motor response
2. Extensor response
3. Abnormal flexion
4. Withdraws
5. Localizes
6. Obeys verbal command

Verbal (V)
1. Nil
2. Incomprehensible sounds
3. Inappropriate words
4. Confused conversation
5. Orientated speech

It can be seen that the GCS assigns a value from 3 to 15. A GCS ≤8 is the definition of coma and is an indication for obtaining a definitive airway (e.g. with an endotracheal tube).

A mild head injury is one associated with a GCS 13–15; a moderate head injury is a GCS 9–12; and a severe head injury is a GCS ≤8.

Pathophysiology

Primary brain injury occurs on impact due to shearing forces that cause tearing of axonal tracts. Primary brain injury accounts for 50% of brain injury deaths. There is little that can be done to minimize the consequences of primary brain injury, and management is thus aimed at preventing secondary effects.

Secondary brain injury may follow primary brain injury because of:

- Extracranial causes – hypoxia from airway obstruction, loss of respiratory drive or pulmonary complications (e.g. acute respiratory distress syndrome) and hypotension from shock due to coexisting injuries. With these conditions, the injured brain loses its ability to regulate its own blood supply (loss of autoregulation) and therefore becomes susceptible to ischaemic damage.
- Intracranial causes – due to raised intracranial pressure (ICP). The Monro–Kellie doctrine explains intracranial compensation for an expanding intracranial space-occupying lesion (SOL): the addition of a SOL (e.g. extradural haematoma, cerebral oedema) within the constant intracranial volume results in the extrusion of an equal volume of CSF and venous blood so that the ICP remains normal. However, when this compensatory mechanism reaches its limit, the ICP will increase exponentially with increased volume of SOL. As CPP = MAP – ICP (cerebral perfusion pressure = mean arterial pressure minus intracranial pressure), when the ICP increases so the CPP will decrease. Hence, the blood flow to the brain becomes compromised and ischaemic damage results. If ICP is allowed to continue to rise, then the medulla oblongata herniates through the tentorium ('coning') with life-threatening consequences as the vital centres are compressed.

Clinical features

The raised ICP compresses the oculomotor nerve (CN III) thus causing papillary dilatation, and compresses the corticospinal tracts – producing motor weakness. The pressure eventually compresses the brainstem ('coning') and the vital cardiorespiratory centre, leading to death.

The increase in ICP leads to a reflex called Cushing's response: the respiratory and heart rates decrease, and the systolic blood pressure increases.

Management

ABC (Airway, Breathing, Circulation) is the priority. Once ABC is stabilized, then D (neurological disability) is assessed using the GCS. It is the trend in GCS, indicating deterioration, stability or improvement, that is important rather than absolute values. Appropriate radiological or MRI imaging can then be performed. In the USA all patients with moderate or severe head injuries should get a CT scan, but in the UK financial restraints prevent this.

Current UK guidelines
Indications for a skull X-ray (some units will do a CT scan)
- Loss of consciousness or a period of amnesia.
- Neurological symptoms and/or signs.
- CSF otorrhoea or rhinorrhoea (CSF coming out of ears or nose).
- Severe scalp injury.
- Suspected penetrating injury with no CT scan available.

Proceed to a CT scan if
- The conscious level as assessed by GCS deteriorates.
- Pupillary signs develop.
- Focal neurological signs develop.
- Skull X-ray reveals a fractured skull (1/4 patients with a fractured skull have evidence of intracranial injury).
- The conscious level does not improve with time.
- The conscious level is difficult to assess, e.g. the patient is intoxicated.
- There is evidence of a penetrating injury.

Indications for hospital admission
- Loss of consciousness >5 min (or amnesia).
- Decreased GCS.
- Skull fracture.
- Neurological symptoms and/or signs.
- Worsening headache, nausea or vomiting.
- Extensive laceration.
- Difficult to assess (e.g. alcohol intoxication).
- No responsible carer at home.
- Other medical conditions (e.g. clotting abnormalities).

A neurosurgical opinion should be sought if there is any suspicion of an intracranial injury. Early endotracheal intubation should be performed on all patients with a severe head injury (GCS ≤8), as it has been shown to reduce the development of secondary brain injury.

Specific management strategies to control ICP, maintain CPP and reduce cerebral metabolic rate for oxygen can be instituted after neurosurgical consultation. However, such advanced measures should be undertaken in an intensive care unit with ICP monitoring facilities.

The use of antibiotics for open skull fractures to prevent meningitis is controversial, as is the administration of corticosteroids to reduce cerebral oedema.

Later complications

Complications require specialist attention and include infection (meningitis, cerebral abscess), which may occur several days after the initial injury. Non-cranial complications may be due to the brain insult or a prolonged ITU (intensive therapy unit) stay. Seizures, gastric ulceration, infection, thromboembolic disease, syndrome of inappropriate antidiuretic hormone secretion (SIADH), disseminated intravascular coagulation (DIC) and intracranial abscess are among the more common sequelae.

Of survivors with brain damage, approximately 50% have permanent after-effects such as paralyses, loss of speech, impaired vision, epilepsy, disturbances of personality or severe mental defects, rendering them disabled for life.

Prognosis

Early neurosurgical consultation, along with rapid treatment to minimize the secondary insult, will improve the prognosis as much as possible. There is little that can be done about the primary brain injury.

Cervical spine injury

Any patient with a serious injury above the clavicle should be assumed to have a coexisting cervical spine injury until this is excluded. Hence, all serious head injury patients should have their cervical spine immobilized according to ATLS (Advanced Trauma Life Support) guidelines (semi-rigid neck collar, sandbags and tape, or in-line immobilization). A cervical spine injury can be excluded in fully conscious patients with normal anteroposterior (AP) and lateral cervical spine X-rays, normal cervical spine examination and normal neurological examination.

All patients with confirmed cervical spine injury should have a neurosurgical opinion.

Dental aspects

The priorities of early management of a patient with maxillofacial injuries, especially if in coma, are:

- Maintain a clear airway.
- Avoid damage to the cervical spine.
- Establish a neurological baseline from the history, consciousness level, examination and pupil reactions.
- Look for other serious injuries; the force necessary to create severe maxillofacial injuries is usually significant enough to cause concomitant injury to the central nervous system, chest, abdomen, pelvis, or extremities, eyes and other bones.

Definitive maxillofacial fracture treatment must usually be delayed until the patient is out of danger unless the fracture hazards the airway, or there is severe haemorrhage. However, early stabilization of grossly displaced or comminuted facial bone fragments may facilitate later management and lessen facial deformity. Soft tissue injuries should be treated early.

Five facts

1. The airway should be protected by endotracheal intubation in patients with severe head injury.
2. The cervical spine should always be immobilized in cases of head injury.
3. The GCS should be monitored regularly for signs of deterioration.
4. A CT scan should be instituted in patients with low or dropping GCS and in patients that are unassessable (e.g. intoxicated).
5. Maxillofacial injuries are often associated with head injury and require careful management of the airway.

Heart failure

Heart failure occurs when the pumping action of the heart (*cardiac output*) is insufficient to meet body demands. The clinical syndrome is of inadequate cardiac output from the left, the right or both sides of the heart, and it may result from a range of pathological processes.

Heart failure is one of the most common causes of hospital admission in elderly people. Most patients with heart failure are over 70 years old.

Clinical features

Left-sided heart failure results in damming of blood back from the left ventricle to the pulmonary circulation with pulmonary hypertension, pulmonary oedema and breathlessness, and the inadequate cardiac output leads to fatigue, decreased exercise tolerance and hypoperfusion of tissues, e.g. renal failure. Shortness of breath is characteristically worsened when laying flat (orthopnoea). In addition, patients may complain of paroxysmal nocturnal dyspnoea (waking up gasping for breath). The severity of shortness of breath associated with heart failure may be graded according to the New York Heart Association (NYHA) grading system summarized in Table 1.

Table 1 New York Heart Association (NYHA) grading system for symptoms of heart failure

NYHA grade	Symptoms	One-year mortality
Grade I	Asymptomatic with ordinary activity	5–10%
Grade II	Slight limitation with physical activity	15%
Grade III	Marked limitation with physical activity	30%
Grade IV	Shortness of breath at rest	50%

Right-sided heart failure causes mainly congestion of the systemic and portal venous systems affecting primarily the liver, gastrointestinal tract, kidneys and subcutaneous tissues. It thus presents with peripheral (dependent) oedema – usually ankle oedema – and fatigue. The liver is usually enlarged (hepatomegaly) due to passive congestion, causing abdominal discomfort and, in severe cardiac failure, raised portal venous pressure also leads to the escape of large amounts of fluid into the peritoneal cavity (ascites).

The patient may also experience features of ischaemic heart disease such as stable angina, acute coronary syndrome and arrhythmias (see chapter on ischaemic heart disease).

Signs of heart failure thus include:

- shortness of breath
- cyanosis (peripheral or central)

- raised jugulo-venous pressure (JVP)
- displacement of the apex beat due to cardiomegaly
- bi-basal course crackles in lungs (indicating pulmonary oedema)
- reduced air entry at the lung bases (indicating bilateral pleural effusions)
- pitting oedema in legs
- hepatomegaly.

Pathology

In heart failure the contractility of the heart is impaired, which leads to a cascade of compensatory physiological mechanisms which act in the short-term to restore cardiac output:

- tissue hypoperfusion leads to activation of the renin–angiotensin–aldosterone system
- angiotensin II both acts directly and via sympathetic stimulation to cause arteriolar vasoconstriction, and thus increases afterload
- aldosterone produces salt and water retention by the kidney, thus increasing preload
- sympathetic stimulation acts on the heart to increase contractility (positively inotropic) and heart rate (positively chronotropic).

In the long term, the extra strain on the heart produces hypertrophy and dilatation of the ventricles, but also myocyte death, which further impairs myocardial contractility, and therefore increases activation of the compensatory mechanisms. A vicious cycle of gradually falling cardiac output therefore develops.

Aetiology

Heart failure may arise from any of several diseases.

Ischaemic heart disease
Ischaemic heart disease is the most common cause.

Valvular heart disease
Any valvular lesion will decrease the efficiency of the heart as a pump and therefore cause heart failure if severe enough. Myocardial contractility must increase to provide an adequate cardiac output, which leads to hypertrophy.

Hypertensive heart disease
Hypertension increases the myocardial contractility required to maintain cardiac output. Over time, this leads to myocardial hypertrophy and cell death.

Pulmonary disease
Multiple pulmonary emboli, COPD (chronic obstructive pulmonary disease) or bronchiectasis lead to increased vascular resistance, causing isolated right-sided heart failure, called *cor pulmonale*.

High output failure

Conditions leading to a high cardiac output either appropriately (e.g. anaemia, pregnancy) or inappropriately (e.g. thyrotoxicosis) cause compensatory hypertrophy which, in the long term, may damage the myocardium.

Cardiomyopathy

Cardiomyopathy is intrinsic disease of the myocardium, and is usually idiopathic. Important identifiable causes are included in Table 2.

Table 2 Classification of causes of cardiomyopathy

Type of disorder	Example of causes
Toxic	Alcohol
	Drugs, e.g. adriamycin, cyclophosphamide
Metabolic	Haemochromatosis
	Uraemia (renal failure)
Infiltrative	Amyloid
	Sarcoid
	Storage disorders, e.g. Gaucher's disease
Endocrine	Thyrotoxicosis
	Hypothyroidism
	Acromegaly
	Diabetes mellitus
Infective	Viral
	Tuberculosis
Hereditary	Hypertrophic cardiomyopathy
	Muscular dystrophy

Investigations

Heart failure is diagnosed clinically and by chest radiography (cardiomegaly), electrocardiography (ECG) and echocardiography. There may also be abnormal liver and renal function tests, hyponatraemia and alkalosis.

Chest radiography

Chest radiography may show cardiomegaly, pulmonary oedema and/or bilateral pleural effusions.

Electrocardiography

ECG may show changes such as ischaemia (ST depression, T-wave inversion), infarction (ST elevation, abnormal Q waves), ventricular hypertrophy or arrhythmias.

Echocardiogram
An echocardiogram provides accurate information on the heart function and structure and the extent of heart failure. It may be performed via the transthoracic or transoesophageal route.

Management

General measures
A *salt-controlled dietary intake* reduces salt and water retention. *Reduction of weight* in the obese, and *smoking cessation* are also important measures. *Treatment of any underlying cause* is obviously vital.

Drugs
- *Loop diuretics* (e.g. furosemide (frusemide)) are the first-line treatment in symptom control, producing salt and water excretion. However, studies have shown no effect on mortality.
- *Oral nitrates* (e.g. isosorbide mononitrate) act predominantly to dilate veins, reduce preload and help symptom control. Hypotension and increasing pharmacological tolerance is a problem.
- *ACE (angiotensin-converting enzyme) inhibitors* act to reduce the compensatory actions of the renin–angiotensin–aldosterone system, and significantly reduce mortality (by about 30%).
- *Beta-blockers* reduce mortality by decreasing sympathetic stimulation.
- *Spironolactone*, an aldosterone antagonist which acts on the distal renal tubules to reduce compensatory fluid retention, reduces symptoms and decreases mortality.
- *Digoxin* improves symptoms but has no effect on mortality.
- *Hydralazine,* an alpha$_1$-adrenoceptor antagonist, causes arterial vasodilatation to reduce afterload. Hypotension limits its use.
- *Aspirin* and *lipid-lowering drugs* (e.g. statins) should be prescribed in heart failure due to ischaemic heart disease.

Cardiac transplantation
Cardiac transplantation in selected patients with advanced failure can significantly improve quality of life and prolong life for years. In most cases, due to the ease of operative procedure, the heart is transplanted in combination with both lungs.

Dental aspects

The dental chair should be kept in a partially reclining or erect position, since it can be dangerous to lay any patient with left-sided heart failure supine as it will worsen dyspnoea.

For patients with *mild* controlled cardiac failure, routine dental care can usually be provided with little modification. In other circumstances, a medical opinion should be obtained. Emergency dental care should be conservative, principally with analgesics and antibiotics. Adrenaline (epinephrine)-containing local anaesthetics should not be given in large doses to patients taking beta-blockers. Supplemental oxygen should be readily available and cardiac monitoring may be desirable.

Five facts

1. Heart failure is defined as inadequate cardiac output to meet the demands of the body.
2. Common symptoms of heart failure are fatigue, shortness of breath, ankle swelling and exertional angina.
3. Common signs of heart failure are dyspnoea, cyanosis, crackles in the chest (due to pulmonary oedema) and leg swelling.
4. Acute management of heart failure is sitting the patient up, high-flow oxygen, intravenous (IV) furosemide (frusemide) and IV glyceryl trinitrate (GTN).
5. Patients with heart failure should be given dental treatment in an upright position to minimize shortness of breath.

Hernias

A hernia is the protrusion of a viscus (organ) through its normal coverings to an ectopic site. The most common hernias (or herniae) are abdominal hernias. Abdominal contents protrude through their peritoneal coverings, due to weaknesses in the abdominal wall. This may be congenital (e.g. a congenital inguinal hernia due to a persistent processus vaginalis), or acquired due to straining combined with weak muscles (e.g. direct inguinal hernia) or at sites of penetration of normal structures through the abdominal wall (e.g. femoral hernias protruding through the femoral canal) or after an operation (incisional hernias). Even coning, in which the medulla oblongata of the brain protrudes through the foramen magnum, is a type of herniation.

It is important to remember that hernias may mask underlying pathology, causing the rise in intra-abdominal pressure that produced the herniation. It is therefore important to consider such causes: e.g. chronic cough in chronic obstructive pulmonary disease (COPD) patients, constipation, urinary retention, pregnancy and ascites. Failure to treat these underlying causes, as well as the hernia, almost inevitably leads to recurrent herniation.

The common types of abdominal hernias are, in decreasing order of frequency:

1. inguinal
2. femoral
3. para-umbilical
4. incisional
5. divarication of the recti
6. epigastric
7. Spigelian
8. umbilical.

Examination and clinical features

The classical features of a hernia on examination are:

1. Reducible lump – refers to the hernia being able to be pushed back into the abdominal cavity. However, not all hernias are reducible.
2. Cough impulse – the thrill felt by the palpating fingers when the patient coughs. Palpating a cough impulse becomes difficult in large hernias with tight necks.

There is much confusion between the terms 'irreducible', 'incarcerated' and 'strangulated', not least because surgeons often use such terms indiscriminately:

- An *irreducible* hernia is one that cannot be reduced, and is thus 'stuck', usually due to adhesions of its contents to the inner wall of the peritoneal sac.
- An *incarcerated* hernia is one that is irreducible but not strangulated, but since some clinicians equate it to strangulation, this term is best avoided.
- A *strangulated* hernia is one with a tight neck cutting off the blood supply to the contents. Unless relieved, the bowel contained within the hernia will become gangrenous and die, with resulting perforation and peritonitis. Hernias with tight

necks (e.g. femoral) are more likely to suffer strangulation than those with wide necks (e.g. incisional).

When a hernia progresses from being simply irreducible to strangulated, the patient will become systemically unwell, complain of severe colicky abdominal pain and have signs of intestinal obstruction (as the strangulated bowel can no longer function properly). The signs of intestinal obstruction are:

- abdominal pain
- vomiting
- abdominal distension
- absolute constipation (no faeces or flatus)
- tinkling bowel sounds.

The severity of these signs will vary with which part of the intestinal system is obstructed. In some cases, only omentum and not bowel is strangulated and hence these signs are much less marked and the patient is at much lower risk of peritonitis. However, it is a brave clinician who does not assume bowel involvement in strangulated abdominal hernias, as the consequences of error are potentially life-threatening.

Inguinal hernia

1. *Indirect* – the hernia enters the deep (internal) inguinal ring and travels down the inguinal canal before exiting from the superficial (external) ring to present as a groin lump.
2. *Direct* – the hernia pushes through the weak transversus abdominis muscles of the abdominal wall to emerge medial to the deep inguinal ring as a groin lump.

The examination point to differentiate these two hernias is the location of the neck of the hernia (i.e. where the hernia reduces to) in relation to the deep inguinal ring. If, after reduction, the hernia can be controlled by pressure over the deep ring, then the hernia is indirect; if this manoeuvre fails to maintain reduction, then the hernia is direct. The location of the deep ring is consistent in man, being found at the mid-inguinal point (half-way between the anterior superior iliac spine and the pubic symphysis).

However, it is true to say that even experienced surgeons often cannot reliably distinguish indirect and direct hernias clinically. The inferior epigastric artery runs immediately medial to the deep ring and, at operation, indirect hernias can thus be seen to originate lateral to this, whereas direct hernias originate as a medial relation. This is the definitive method for differentiation. In a few cases, however, the hernia is found to have two necks – one lateral and one medial to the inferior epigastric artery. This hernia is thus a combination of the direct and indirect hernia, and has the intraoperative appearance of a bag of trousers; it is thus aptly termed a 'pantaloon hernia'.

It may also be difficult to clinically distinguish an inguinal hernia from a femoral hernia. However, this can be achieved reliably by using the pubic tubercle as an anatomical landmark, which can be located by palpating the pubic symphysis and moving your fingers laterally, or by palpating the adductor magnus tendon when the patient's thigh is externally rotated and following it up to its origin. The neck of a femoral hernia lies below and lateral to the pubic tubercle, whereas that of an inguinal hernia lies above and medial to it. It is important when performing this examination to palpate the neck of the hernia and not its sac, as this can spread out anywhere in the region.

Indirect hernias are due to a congenital weakness in the abdominal wall at a specific anatomical location, and thus need elective surgical repair to prevent obstruction or strangulation. Direct hernias are due to a general acquired weakness in the abdominal wall, usually as a result of age, and thus direct hernias affect a much older age group than indirect hernias, which are common in young and middle-aged adult men. Direct hernias have a low risk of obstruction and strangulation due to their wide necks and are thus repaired only if causing discomfort or cosmetic problems to the patient.

Femoral hernia

This hernia protrudes the femoral canal, which is an anatomical space about 1.5 cm long. Hence, any femoral hernia has a tight neck and is more susceptible than an inguinal hernia to strangulation. Due to the wider pelvis in females, femoral hernias are much more common in women than men. The risk of strangulation means than asymptomatic femoral hernias should be surgically repaired electively within a month, and symptomatic femoral hernias repaired on the next available operating list. Strangulated hernias need immediate repair to prevent perforation and peritonitis.

Differential diagnosis of a groin lump

1. Inguinal hernia (indirect and direct).
2. Femoral hernia.
3. Saphena varix (varicose veins of the great saphenous vein).
4. Femoral aneurysm.
5. Inguinal lymphadenopathy (secondary to infection or malignancy).
6. Psoas abscess.
7. Ectopic testis.
8. Lipoma.
8. Sebaceous cyst.

The easiest way to remember this list is to think of the structures in the inguinal region anatomically (skin – sebaceous cyst; subcutaneous tissues – lipoma; inguinal canal – inguinal hernia, lymphadenopathy; femoral canal – femoral hernia; great saphenous vein – saphena varix; femoral artery – femoral aneurysm; and psoas muscle – psoas abscess).

Other abdominal hernias

- *Para-umbilical* – protrude from around the umbilicus and have a narrow neck making strangulation likely. Hence, early surgical repair is advised.
- *Incisional* – protrudes from the site of the operative scar and thus has a wide neck and a low risk of strangulation. Repair is therefore not essential.

- *Divarication of the recti (ventral hernia)* – protrudes from the gap between the two rectus muscles in elderly, cachectic patients, and usually requires no treatment.
- *Epigastric* – protrudes through a defect in the midline linea alba and usually contains only fat or omentum.
- *Spigelian* – protrudes through the linea semilunaris (outermost border of the rectus) and usually requires surgical repair.
- *Umbilical* – protrudes through a defect in the umbilical scar, and is thus a congenital defect, common in babies of African descent. These hernias usually resolve spontaneously as the defect closes by the end of the first year of life.
- Hernias can also rarely occur at other sites, such as through the obturator foramen (obturator), greater sciatic foramen (gluteal), lesser sciatic foramen (sciatic) and inferior lumbar triangle (lumbar).

Treatment of abdominal hernias

Predisposing factors that increase intra-abdominal pressure have to be managed before any surgical repair is attempted. Surgical repair is typically by mesh repair and can be performed by an open or laparoscopic technique, with low rates of recurrence and postoperative infection. With hernias at low risk of strangulation where the patient is not surgically fit, large hernias can be controlled by means of wearing a truss.

Dental aspects

There is no immediate dental relevance, unless the dental staff themselves have a hernia!

Five facts

1. A hernia is a protrusion of an organ through its normal coverings.
2. Raised intra-abdominal pressure (e.g. COPD, constipation) can predispose to hernia.
3. Inguinal hernias are the commonest type of abdominal hernia in both sexes.
4. Femoral hernias are commoner in women than in men, and are more likely to get strangulated than other types of hernia.
5. Elective repair is usually with a mesh.

HIV and AIDS

The main activity of the immune system is protection against infections. The immune responses depends on immunocytes – lymphocytes and macrophages producing humoral (antibody – mainly B cell) or cell-mediated (mainly T cell) responses, but often both. Cell-mediated immunity is particularly important in defence against viruses and fungi, some intracellular bacteria such as mycobacteria, in delayed hypersensitivity and in defences against cancer cells. CD4 cells are crucial cells in cell-mediated immunity, and are mainly helper T cells important in antigen processing and other immune functions. Healthy adults usually have CD4+ T-cell counts of >1000 per cubic millimetre (microlitre) of blood. Human immunodeficiency virus (HIV) is an RNA retrovirus which damages the body's cellular immunity, mainly damaging CD4 cells.

HIV versus AIDS

Infection with HIV is termed *HIV infection*, and this can be asymptomatic for many months or years. When clinical disease appears, the term *HIV disease* is used. Individuals with HIV infection may progress to develop *acquired immunodeficiency syndrome (AIDS)*. Under the 1993 Centers for Disease Control (CDC) case definition, AIDS is diagnosed in an HIV-positive individual when the individual's CD4+ cell count has fallen below 200 cells per microlitre, when CD4+ cells account for fewer than 14% of all lymphocytes or when an AIDS-defining illness is present (see below).

Worldwide impact of disease

HIV/AIDS has become the highest profile disease and one of the most important diseases worldwide since its recognition in 1981 and is a communicable disease with an enormous array of clinical manifestations. It is also a disease with a huge social impact; therefore, a good understanding of HIV/AIDS is necessary for all health professionals.

Epidemiology

In 2004, the World Heath Organization (WHO) estimated that about 35 million people were infected worldwide. AIDS is the main cause of death in many countries in the developing world, many of which are in Africa. The rising incidence of AIDS in such poor countries is a major cause of economic underdevelopment.

Pathology

HIV is an RNA lentivirus. HIV-1 and HIV-2 cause disease, but HIV-1 is much more prevalent. HIV causes persistent infection of, and destruction of, CD4+ T lymphocytes.

Two factors account for the virulence of HIV. First, HIV is able to mutate its genome and therefore evade immune attack. Secondly, a minority of HIV virions may remain dormant and incorporated into the genome of host lymphocytes and may only be reactivated after a prolonged period, therefore evading immune defences.

Routes of transmission

- *Sexual contact* is the most common route of HIV transmission. Education and the practice of barrier contraception reduces sexual transmission. Anal sex has a higher risk of infection than vaginal sex. Thus, unprotected and homosexual intercourse are the most common routes of transmission. The risk of transmission via saliva is very small. Saliva contains some protective factors.
- *Intravenous (IV) drug abuse* is a big problem, particularly with the practice of needle-sharing among drug users. Public health initiatives to provide clean, free needles have reduced this route of transmission.
- *Vertical transmission* is where an infected pregnant mother passes HIV to her fetus. If the baby is not infected at birth, transmission may occur during breast-feeding.
- *Blood transfusions* were an important route of HIV transmission before routine screening of blood products for HIV was adopted in the 1980s and, as a result, many haemophiliac individuals at that time became HIV positive. The risk of HIV infection from blood is now extremely low in the developed world.
- *Needlestick injuries* and infection via mucosal surfaces such as the eyes are important but rare modes of transmission and can cause occupational transmission in health professionals.

Clinical features

Primary HIV infection
Primary HIV infection may go unrecognized but 2–4 weeks after infection, a non-specific febrile illness resembling glandular fever is usual. Myalgia, a maculopapular rash and generalized lymphadenopathy may all occur. During this period, there is a transient drop in the CD4 count, and a rise in the CD8 count.

Asymptomatic phase (HIV infection)
In this condition, there may be mild, self-limiting febrile illnesses, and generalized lymphadenopathy. The CD4 count is normal and the CD8 count is raised.

Intermediate phase (HIV disease)
'Non-opportunistic' infections (e.g. salmonella, shingles) increase in incidence and severity. The CD4 count starts to drop, but the CD8 count remains within normal limits.

Acquired immunodeficiency syndrome
Less pathogenic, opportunist infections cause disease. The occurrence of AIDS-defining illnesses heralds the diagnosis of AIDS. The CD4 count drops further, and the CD8 count eventually drops as well.

Examples of AIDS-defining illnesses are:

- cytomegalovirus (CMV) retinitis
- *Pneumocystis carinii* pneumonia (PCP)
- miliary or extrapulmonary tuberculosis (TB) – sometimes multi-drug resistant

- atypical mycobacterioses: e.g. *Mycobacterium avium-intracellulare* (MAI)
- Kaposi's sarcoma
- non-Hodgkin's lymphomas, primary cerebral lymphoma
- cyptococcal meningitis
- oral and oesophageal candidiasis
- cerebral toxoplasmosis
- progressive multifocal leukoencephalopathy (PMLE).

Complications of AIDS

Respiratory

Tuberculosis
Immunodeficiency can lead to reactivation of old, dormant TB and also predisposes the individual to new infection if exposed.

Pneumocystis carinii
This fungal infection may cause pneumonia with shortness of breath on exertion, dry cough and fever. Oxygen desaturation on exertion is a characteristic finding. Chest X-ray appearances normally show perihilar shadowing, but may show other patterns of consolidation, cavitation and infiltration, or even be entirely normal. Microscopy of sputum or bronchial washings with Indian ink will reveal cysts and trophozoites. Treatment is with co-trimoxazole.

Gastrointestinal tract

Candidiasis
Candidiasis commonly occurs in the mouth, but may be found in the oesophagus. It causes dysphagia, and is treated with an oral antifungal agent such as fluconazole.

Oral hairy leukoplakia
Oral hairy leukoplakia presents as white plaques on the tongue. It is strongly associated with Epstein–Barr virus (EBV). It is usually asymptomatic.

Cytomegalovirus
Gastrointestinal infection (GI) most commonly affects the oesophagus and colon. Treatment is with ganciclovir.

Cryptosporidiosis
Cryptosporidiosis is a protozoal infection which may infect the large or small bowel to cause chronic diarrhoea with watery stools and malabsorption. Diagnosis is by stool microscopy and/or duodenal biopsy.

Other gastrointestinal infections
Other GI infections which may cause diarrhoeal illness in AIDS include those caused by *Mycobacterium avium-intracellulare*, *Microsporidium*, *Giardia*, *Shigella* and *Salmonella*.

Central nervous system

Meningitis
Meningitis may occur secondary to TB and fungi such as *Cryptococcus* and *Candida* (see chapter on meningitis).

Toxoplasma gondii
Toxoplasma gondii is a protozoan which tends to form focal brain lesions (which may have ring-enhancement with IV contrast on computed tomography (CT)) and may present with headache, confusion, drowsiness and seizures.

Primary CNS lymphoma
Primary CNS lymphoma is closely associated with EBV and typically produces a single periventricular lesion, which may have ring-enhancement on CT.

Progressive multifocal leukoencephalopathy
PMLE is an invariably fatal type of encephalitis caused by JC virus infection.

HIV infection
HIV infection of the brain parenchyma can itself cause dementia.

Skin

Kaposi's sarcoma
Kaposi's sarcoma is a cutaneous neoplasm associated with human herpesvirus 8 (HHV-8), which appears as multiple red-purple papules or nodules. Localized lesions may be treated by excision and local chemotherapy/radiotherapy and metastatic disease is treated with systemic chemotherapy.

Herpes simplex virus and varicella zoster virus
Herpes simplex virus (HSV) and varicella zoster virus (VZV) dormant infection may reactivate to cause herpes labialis or shingles, respectively. Treatment is aciclovir or valaciclovir.

Eye
CMV, toxoplasma, TB and candidiasis may all cause retinitis.

HIV infections
Infections in HIV according to CD4 count (cells per microlitre) are given in Table 1.

Investigations

HIV serology
The most common HIV test assays the antibody titre to a specific HIV antigen in serum. Note that it may take up to 6 months for an individual to seroconvert. The ELISA (enzyme-linked immunosorbent assay) test is used, followed by a confirmatory Western blot assay.

Table 1 Infections in HIV according to CD4 count

CD4 count (cells per microlitre)	Commonly associated infections
>500	Vaginal candidiasis
<500	Pulmonary TB
	HSV, VZV
	Salmonella, Shigella
	Kaposi's sarcoma
	Oral candidiasis
	Oral hairy leukoplakia
<200	PCP
	Cryptosporidium, Microsporidium
	Oesophageal candidiasis
<100	CNS disease
	Mycobacterium avium-intracellulare
<50	CMV retinitis

CD4 count
CD4 count is measured in order to monitor the extent of immunosuppression, and response to treatment.

HIV viral load
The polymerase chain reaction (PCR) may be used to measure the number of viral copies in the serum. It gives an indication of disease progression.

Management

Confidentiality
It is particularly important to maintain strict confidentiality with patients with HIV because of the social stigma the diagnosis causes (remember the film 'Philadelphia'?).

Support/counselling
Affected individuals must be offered specialized counselling before any HIV test is done.

Drug treatment
Anti-HIV drugs include:

- *Nucleoside analogue reverse transcriptase inhibitors*, e.g. zidovudine (AZT), didanosine (ddI), prevent further lengthening of the DNA strand, and therefore inhibit viral replication.
- *Non-nucleoside analogue reverse transcriptase inhibitors*, e.g. nevirapine, bind to HIV reverse transcriptase and inhibit its function.

- *Protease inhibitors (PI)*, e.g. indinavir, prevent post-translational cleavage of precursor proteins into the actual proteins needed for virion synthesis.

A combination, usually of three anti-HIV drugs (*triple therapy*) is always used, in order to combat drug resistance. This type of drug regime generally includes a protease inhibitor and is referred to as highly active anti-retroviral treatment (HAART); a typical regime is AZT, didanosine and indinavir. The decision of when to initiate HAART is difficult and should balance the need to treat disease before immunosuppression becomes too profound, against the significant adverse effects of HAART. However, HAART should always be commenced if the CD4 count is <200. Current practice is to commence HAART if the CD4 count is <350, dependent on viral load.

Contact tracing

HIV is a notifiable disease, and previous sexual contacts must be traced and tested for HIV. If the patient's partner is uninfected, barrier sexual intercourse must be practised.

Treatment of other sexually transmitted diseases (STDs)

People who get HIV from sexual contact should be screened for other STDs, e.g. chlamydia, warts, gonorrhoea and syphilis (see chapter on sexually transmitted diseases).

Post-exposure prophylaxis

Post-exposure prophylaxis (PEP) is by short-term anti-retroviral treatment to minimize the risk of HIV infection after potential exposure. The risk of transmission of HIV from an infected patient through an open-bore needlestick is less than 1%. The risk of transmission from exposure to infected fluids or tissues is believed to be lower than exposure to infected blood. Regular supervision in health care settings can help to deter or reduce risk of occupational hazards in the workplace.

If injury or contamination results in exposure to HIV-infected material, post-exposure counselling, treatment, follow-up and care should be provided. First aid should be given immediately after the injury. Wounds and skin sites exposed to blood or body fluids should be washed with soap and water, and mucous membranes flushed with water. The exposure should be evaluated immediately by the occupational health team for its potential to transmit HIV infection. PEP for HIV should be provided as soon as possible when exposure to a person with HIV has occurred (or it is likely that the source person is infected with HIV). A combination of zidovudine, lamivudine and indinavir or better, nelfinavir, for 4 weeks may be recommended.

Dental aspects

The chief occupational risk of acquiring infection is as a result of injury by a sharp instrument, particularly a local anaesthetic needle which can contain a significant amount of contaminated fluid. Although needlestick injuries can transmit the virus, infection among health care personnel caring for HIV-infected patients is rare despite reports of many such injuries. It is unethical to withhold treatment from any patient on the basis of a moral judgement that the patient's activities or lifestyle might have contributed to the condition for which treatment was being sought.

HIV does appear to have been transmitted within health care facilities on rare occasions. One dentist with HIV infection in Florida, USA, appears to have transmitted it to at least 6 patients as a consequence of invasive dental procedures. That the dentist was the source of the infection was suggested by the fact that the strain of the virus was the same. The precise mode of transmission remains uncertain as the dentist has since died. An outbreak of 14 cases of HIV infection was discovered by chance among haemodialysis patients at a university hospital in Bucaramanga, Colombia, and seems most likely to have been transmitted by contaminated dental instruments.

Many other studies, however, have shown no evidence of any transmission of HIV from HIV-infected dentists to patients.

The majority of patients with HIV disease have experienced head and neck and oral manifestations at some time, particularly when the CD4 cell count is low. Cervical lymphadenopathy is an almost invariable feature of HIV disease and AIDS. Oral candidiasis is common, and frequently associated with oesophageal candidiasis. Infections with HSV, VZV, CMV, Epstein–Barr virus, human herpes virus 6 (HHV-6) and HHV-8 are common. Mycobacterial oral ulcers and oral histoplasmosis or cryptococcosis, as well as sinusitis, gingivitis or periodontitis, may be seen. Aphthous-like ulcers may be seen. Chronic parotitis is common in children with HIV, and virtually pathognomonic. Kaposi's sarcoma and lymphomas may be seen in the mouth.

Further reading

UK Health Departments. *HIV post-exposure prophylaxis: guidance from the UK Chief Medical Officers' Expert Advisory Group on AIDS.* July 2000.

Five facts

1. HIV is a viral infection of the immune system (mainly CD4+ lymphocytes), causing progressive immunosuppression.
2. The main modes of transmission of HIV are sexual, vertical and via blood (transfusion, intravenous drug use (IVDU) or needlestick injury).
3. AIDS is defined as when an individual with HIV develops an AIDS-defining illness, or the CD4+ count is <200 cells per microlitre or <14% of lymphocytes.
4. After a needlestick injury, the occupational health team or local casualty department should be contacted immediately to start post-exposure prophylaxis.
5. In AIDS, oral infections such as candida, herpes, varicella zoster, cytomegalovirus, mycobacterial oral ulcers, oral histoplasmosis and cryptococcosis may be seen as may tumours such as Kaposi's sarcoma or lymphoma.

Hypertension

Blood pressure is necessary to perfuse the organs of the body with blood, so is vital to the sustainment of life. The normal blood pressure (BP) is 120 mmHg systolic and 80 mmHg diastolic. Hypertension describes the state of chronically raised blood pressure, and is commonly defined as a BP in excess of 140/90 mmHg; about 20% of the population are, by this measure, hypertensive.

Epidemiology

Hypertension is common and its incidence increases with age. There is considerable ethnic variation, and Afro-Caribbean individuals are at a much greater risk of hypertension than Caucasians.

Clinical features

Hypertension is a mostly asymptomatic condition in the early stages, but may lead to several complications, particularly cardiovascular, renal and ocular. If untreated, hypertension shortens life by 10–20 years. Hypertension per se normally gives no symptoms but there may be symptoms and signs of the complications of hypertension.

Some common clinical features thus include:

- *Cardiovascular* – left ventricular hypertrophy (evidenced by displacement of the apex beat), ischaemic heart disease and heart failure.
- *Cerebrovascular* – the incidence of ischaemic stroke is increased due to the formation of atherosclerotic plaques. Hypertension also increases the incidence of subarachnoid and intracerebral haemorrhage.
- *Peripheral vascular disease* – aortic dissection, aneurysm formation and peripheral vascular insufficiency are all associated with atherosclerosis promoted by hypertension.
- *Renal* – there may be evidence of hypertensive renal disease in the form of oliguria or proteinuria.
- *Ocular* – retinopathy is an important clinical feature of hypertension. It may be graded according to findings on fundoscopy, in ascending order of severity of disease:
  - Grade I = silver wiring appearance of blood vessels
  - Grade II = Grade I + arteriovenous nipping
  - Grade III = Grade II + cotton wool spots and flame haemorrhages
  - Grade IV = Grade III + papilloedema (swelling of the optic disc).

Malignant/accelerated hypertension is a rare condition of rapidly progressive hypertension with end-organ damage. It is characterized by Grade III or IV retinopathy, proteinuria, and/or hypertensive encephalopathy (which may present with drowsiness, confusion and fits).

Aetiopathogenesis

The aetiology for hypertension is unclear (idiopathic) in most cases (primary hypertension) but a variety of specific conditions may cause hypertension in the minority (secondary hypertension). The renin–angiotensin–aldosterone (RAA) system has a central role in secondary hypertension.

Primary hypertension

Primary hypertension is thought to be due to an interaction between genetic and environmental factors. The wide racial variation in incidence (much higher incidence in Afro-Caribbean individuals) illustrates the genetic importance. Environmental factors thought to be important include high salt and alcohol intake and a low fruit and vegetable diet.

Secondary hypertension

The causes of secondary hypertension may be classified as follows.

Cardiac
Coarctation of the aorta
Coarctation of the aorta is a congenital narrowing in the aorta, most commonly just distal to the origin of the left subclavian artery. Blood pressure is raised proximal to the narrowing, but may be normal or low distal to the narrowing. Associated features include weak femoral pulses, radiofemoral delay and a systolic murmur heard loudest over the site of the coarctation.

Aortic incompetence
Clinical features such as an early diastolic murmur heard best in the aortic area, as well as a wide pulse pressure and heart failure, may be seen.

Renal (see chapter on renal disease)
Renal artery stenosis
Renal artery stenosis is a narrowing of one or more of the renal arteries, which leads to reduced blood flow to the affected kidney and hypertension. A renal bruit may be heard over the affected kidney.

Polycystic kidney disease
Polycystic kidney disease is a group of genetic diseases characterized by bilateral cystic enlargement of the kidneys. It presents with hypertension, chronic renal failure or abdominal masses.

Chronic renal failure
Chronic renal failure, particularly glomerulonephritis, is characterized by hypertension, due to impaired glomerular filtration.

Endocrine (see chapter on adrenal disorders)
Cushing's syndrome
Cushing's syndrome results from the overproduction of glucocorticoids (mainly cortisol) by the adrenal cortex, stimulated either by a pituitary adenoma, an adrenal adenoma, or ectopic ACTH (adrenocorticotrophic hormone) secretion from a

tumour. Excess glucocorticoids may produce hypertension, centripetal fat distribution, moon facies, hirsutism, acne and proximal muscle wasting.

Conn's syndrome
Conn's syndrome results from the overproduction of mineralocorticoids (mainly aldosterone) by the adrenal cortex, normally caused by an adrenal adenoma. Excess aldosterone leads to sodium and water retention via its effect on the kidney, which causes hypertension.

Phaeochromocytoma
Phaeochromocytoma is a neoplasm of the adrenal medulla, which leads to the overproduction of catecholamines. Patients often experience paroxysmal palpitations and anxiety.

Congenital adrenal hyperplasia
Congenital adrenal hyperplasia is a deficiency in 11β-hydroxylase or 17-hydroxylase, leading to hypertension via excess formation of the mineralocorticoid 11-deoxycorticosterone.

Others
Other endocrine causes include pregnancy, acromegaly and thyrotoxicosis.

Drugs
Secondary hypertension is also caused by drugs such as ciclosporin and corticosteroids.

Investigations

Serial blood pressure measurements provide the simplest method of diagnosis, but BP taken in a clinical environment may not always accurately represent the true BP of the patient in their home environment since anxiety causes a rise. *Continuous ambulatory BP measurement* provides an accurate record of the BP of the patient over a 24-hour period. However, it is not widely available.

Screening for end-organ effects of hypertension
It is important to look for end-organ effects of hypertension. An electrocardiogram (ECG) is used to detect left ventricular hypertrophy, as well as ischaemic heart disease. Echocardiography is excellent for assessment of left ventricular hypertrophy and cardiac function. Measurement of serum urea and electrolytes and urine dipstix will detect renal impairment and proteinuria, respectively.

Screening for secondary causes of hypertension
Although most cases of hypertension are primary, detection of a secondary cause is important since treatment of that cause may cure the patient of hypertension.

- *Urea and electrolytes*: to detect renal impairment.
- *Ultrasound of kidneys:* to detect renal structural disease (e.g. polycystic kidneys or obstructive nephropathy).

- *24-hour urine collection* with measurement of urinary cortisol and catecholamines, to screen for Cushing's disease and phaeochromocytoma.
- *Chest radiograph*: cardiomegaly may indicate left ventricular hypertrophy caused by hypertension. Rib notching and an abnormal aortic arch may be present in coarctation.
- *Plasma renin/aldosterone measurement*: to detect Conn's syndrome.
- *Thyroid function tests:* to detect thyrotoxicosis.

Screening for other cardiovascular risk factors
Hypertension is a major risk factor for cardiovascular disease. It is therefore vital to address other risk factors such as diabetes mellitus, hyperlipidaemia, obesity and smoking (see chapter on ischaemic heart disease).

Management

The important aspects of management of hypertension are a change in lifestyle (Table 1) and the reduction of coexistent cardiovascular risk factors, such as diabetes mellitus, obesity and hyperlipidaemia.

Table 1 Lifestyle risk factors modifying hypertension

Factors raising BP	*Factors lowering BP*
Obesity	No obesity
High dietary salt intake	Low salt intake
Excess alcohol	Low alcohol intake
Smoking	Cessation of smoking
Physical inactivity	Physical activity
Stress/anxiety	Relaxation
	High fibre diet
	Omega-3 fatty acids
	Fruit and vegetables
	Supplemental potassium

However, the mainstay of treatment of hypertension remains pharmacological, in the form of four main classes of antihypertensive agent. It is often a case of trial and error with the uses of one or more of these classes of drug before adequate BP control is achieved.

Beta-blockers
Beta-blockers such as atenolol inhibit beta-adrenergic receptors in the heart and vasculature. They therefore dilate blood vessels, and reduce heart contractility (negatively inotropic) and rate. Newer beta-blockers such as bisoprolol are cardio-selective, and therefore act predominantly on the heart. Beta-blockers are contraindicated in asthma and severe heart failure.

Angiotensin-converting enzyme (ACE) inhibitors

ACE inhibitors act by inhibiting ACE, which normally catalyses the conversion of angiotensin (AT) I to AT II. AT II stimulates production of renin (and therefore aldosterone). *AT II receptor antagonists* specifically inhibit the action of AT II, but do not affect bradykinin metabolism, unlike ACE inhibitors. Therefore, they do not cause the side effect of coughing, unlike ACE inhibitors. These drugs are contraindicated in renal impairment, renal artery stenosis and pregnancy.

Calcium channel antagonists

Calcium channel antagonists such as nifedipine and amlodipine act to directly cause vasodilatation. Verapamil is cardioselective, and is negatively inotropic. Their side effects include palpitations and flushing. They are contraindicated in heart failure.

Thiazide diuretics

Thiazide diuretics, e.g. bendroflumethiazide, act via diuresis and other incompletely understood mechanisms to reduce blood pressure. They may cause postural hypotension and gout.

Other anti-hypertensive drugs

Other anti-hypertensive drugs that are less commonly used include *alpha-adrenergic antagonists*, e.g. prazosin, and *centrally acting drugs*, e.g. methyldopa.

Dental aspects

It is essential to avoid anxiety and pain, since endogenous adrenaline (epinephrine) released in response to pain or fear may induce dysrhythmias. Raising the patient suddenly from the supine position may cause postural hypotension and loss of consciousness if the patient is using antihypertensive drugs.

An aspirating syringe should be used to give a local anaesthetic, since adrenaline (epinephrine) in the anaesthetic given intravenously may (theoretically) increase hypertension and precipitate arrhythmias. Some non-steroidal anti-inflammatory drugs (NSAIDs) such as indometacin, ibuprofen and naproxen can reduce the efficacy of antihypertensive agents.

There are no recognized oral manifestations of hypertension. Antihypertensive drugs can sometimes cause effects such as xerostomia, salivary gland swelling or pain, lichenoid reactions, erythema multiforme, angio-oedema, gingival hyperplasia, sore mouth or paraesthesiae.

Five facts

1. Hypertension is defined as a blood pressure in excess of 140/90 mmHg.
2. Complications are cardiovascular, cerebrovascular, peripheral vascular, renal and ocular.
3. Its aetiology may be primary (most cases) or secondary.
4. The four main classes of drug used to treat hypertension are beta-blockers, ACE inhibitors, calcium channel antagonists and thiazide diuretics.
5. Raising the patient suddenly from the supine position may cause postural hypotension and loss of consciousness if the patient is using antihypertensive drugs.

Infection control and MRSA

Infection control

Infection control is of prime importance in clinical practice. It is essential to the safety of patients, families and staff. Every member of staff must receive training in all aspects of infection control, including decontamination of instruments and equipment, and a policy must be adhered to at all times. All staff must be immunized against hepatitis B and a record of their hepatitis B seroconversion held by the employer. For those who do not seroconvert, or cannot be immunized, medical advice and counselling should be given. In these cases it may be necessary to restrict their clinical activities.

Protective clothing, gloves, eyewear and masks must be worn during all operative procedures. Protective clothing worn in the surgery should not be worn outside the premises. Before donning gloves, hands must be washed. Any glove that becomes damaged must be replaced and a new pair of gloves must be used for each patient. All instruments that have been potentially contaminated must be sterilized. Single-use items must not be decontaminated and reused. Needles, scalpel blades, LA (local anaesthetic) vials, burs, matrix bands, etc., must be disposed of in a yellow sharps container. All clinical waste must be placed in appropriate sacks or bins and securely fastened when three-quarters full, stored in a designated area and disposed of safely.

In the event of an inoculation injury, the wound should be allowed to bleed, washed thoroughly under running water and covered with a waterproof dressing. The incident should be immediately discussed with, and advice on post-exposure prophylaxis obtained from, the occupational health physician.

Surgical infections

Antibiotics have been in use for more than 50 years and many organisms are now resistant to the older agents. Overuse of antibiotics encourages the development of microbial resistance, destroys the normal flora, thus making the patient more susceptible to colonization with hospital organisms (nosocomial infections), and predisposes to *Clostridium difficile* infection, which can lead to pseudomembranous colitis.

Methicillin-resistant *Staphylococcus aureus* (MRSA), vancomycin-resistant *S. aureus* (VRSA), vancomycin-resistant enterococci (VRE) and multi-resistant *Pseudomonas aeruginosa* are of concern since they can infect surgical sites and have now become important nosocomial infections.

MRSA

MRSA, popularly termed the 'superbug' by most tabloid newspapers, is resistant to methicillin, which was a precursor of flucloxacillin and is no longer used in clinical practice. The importance of methicillin (meticillin) resistance is that it predicts resistance to all *beta-lactam* antibiotics (e.g. penicillin, flucloxacillin) and also all cephalosporins. MRSA is of particular concern in the management of patients with burns, skin grafts and flaps, and prostheses, where tissue penetration of the antibiotic is of paramount importance, and where an infection may lead to the need to remove a prosthesis or graft failure.

Most strains of MRSA have now acquired resistance to other classes of antibiotic as well, and thus the term methicillin-resistant *S. aureus* is being replaced by the term multi-resistant *S. aureus*. The newer strains of MRSA may also express virulence factors which lead to rapid dissemination within a hospital. A typical example is the strain EMRSA-16, which caused a major outbreak in Kettering in 1991 and has since spread to most hospitals in the UK. MRSA infection is also extremely difficult to treat; oral therapy with rifampicin plus fusidic acid is hepatotoxic and has been replaced with linezolid.

Glycopeptide antibiotics such as vancomycin and teicoplanin are the most commonly used intravenous treatments for MRSA, but these are more toxic than most other antibacterials, penetrate less well into abscesses, infected bone and cerebrospinal fluid, and are more expensive.

Another concern is the emergence of VRSA, currently mainly in the USA and Japan. It may be that *S. aureus* will be untreatable in the near future, and that we will have to find new strategies to combat this devastating infection.

Control of MRSA and other resistant organisms

The main mode of spread of resistant organisms is on the hands of health care workers. This hand carriage is usually transient and the chain of infection can be prevented by hand washing between each patient examined. MRSA can also survive for hours on hard surfaces, so maintaining a clean clinical environment is also vital. Hands should be washed either with soap/chlorhexidine/povidone-iodine solutions and water or, if the hands are not visibly soiled, with alcohol rubs or gels.

Another way of controlling MRSA is to identify colonized patients or staff (see below), allowing precautionary measures to be taken to prevent the spread of the organism to other people, and also to reduce the risk of clinical infection in patients planned for high-risk surgery (e.g. vascular graft surgery, prosthetic orthopaedic surgery). Colonization is identified by taking swabs from the nose, throat and perineum. Such patients are usually asymptomatic and do not require systemic antibiotic treatment unless they develop signs of clinical infection. However, attempts to eradicate MRSA in colonized patients using standard preoperative prophylaxis (e.g. chlorhexidine wash) should be made. This will often fail in the presence of foreign bodies such as percutaneous feeding tubes and persisting wounds, in which situation topical agents (e.g. mupirocin) are preferred as well as careful attention to intra- and post-operative aseptic technique.

If there is evidence of an outbreak in a unit, staff may also be screened in case they are carriers; however, this should be done only at the request of the infection control team.

Other principles of infection control in the case of resistant organisms

Once patients have been found to be colonized with a significant multi-resistant organism, they should enter 'source' isolation, such as being nursed in a side room.

All staff and visitors must wear disposable gloves and aprons when in physical contact with the patient with MRSA. Studies have shown white coats to be a portal of infection, and they should be removed before entering the room. The number of personnel in contact with the patient should be limited as much as possible.

Preoperative patients known to be colonized with multi-resistant organisms should generally be operated on at the end of the surgical list so that the theatre can be cleaned thoroughly afterwards and presents no risk to the next patient. The same applies to visits to other departments such as radiology, physiotherapy, etc., where again the infected patient should be the last case of the day. Avoidance of ward transfers and other unnecessary movements is of utmost importance.

Antibiotics should only be used in cases of clinical infection or as part of a preoperative prophylaxis policy as defined by a microbiologist.

Dental aspects

Infection control is particularly important in maxillofacial surgery and in the immunocompromised patient.

Five facts

1. All staff must be immunized against hepatitis B.
2. The risk of contracting HIV from a needlestick injury is minimal, but in some cases PEP (post-exposure prophylaxis) may be advised.
3. Hand washing is the single most important preventative measure against infection.
4. Immunocompromised patients are more susceptible to infection.
5. All staff should be screened if there is an MRSA outbreak, and strict isolation procedures should be employed.

Infective endocarditis

Infective endocarditis (IE) is infection of the endocardium (inner layer of the heart), and in particular of the heart valves. IE is a serious condition that is associated with a high rate of mortality if untreated.

Infective endocarditis predominantly affects natural heart valves (native valve endocarditis) sometimes damaged by diseases such as rheumatic carditis, but can also involve prosthetic heart valves or congenital heart defects (such as coarctation of the aorta or ductus arteriosus).

Classification

The main types of infective endocarditis are:

1. *Acute bacterial endocarditis* – very aggressive, short time course. Normal (undamaged) valves are affected, and *Staphylococcus aureus* is the main pathogen.
2. *Native valve endocarditis (subacute bacterial endocarditis)* – which affects natural valves, typically in situations where there is abnormal turbulence of the blood flow caused by valve damage/defect. *Streptococcus viridans,* an upper respiratory tract and oral cavity commensal bacterium, is the most common cause of IE. Cardiac valves already damaged by infective endocarditis are especially susceptible.
3. *Prosthetic valve endocarditis* – infection of cardiac prostheses, especially valves.

Pathology

In general, IE results from two main predisposing factors – bacteraemia and a cardiac lesion where there is turbulent blood flow.

Platelets and fibrin deposits accumulate at sites where there is turbulent blood flow over damaged valves (non-bacterial thrombotic endocarditis). These sterile vegetations can thereafter be readily infected during bacteraemias, resulting in infective endocarditis. *Streptococcus viridans* is the most common organism involved.

Although IE may occur in anyone, certain groups of people are more at risk:

- *Congenital heart defects* predispose to IE, particularly if they have a high pressure gradient across them (e.g. ventricular septal defect).
- *Acquired heart disease* sometimes predisposes to IE, mainly if there is scarring, e.g. after rheumatic carditis following rheumatic fever.
- *Prosthetic heart valves* and *central venous catheters* provide an excellent site for seeding of any blood-borne infection, due to their prosthetic surface. *Staphylococcus epidermidis* infection is the main cause of prosthesis-associated infection, e.g. prosthetic heart valve, or central venous catheter infection at the time of its placement. It forms a biofilm around any prosthetic material which physically protects it from the host immune system. *Streptococcus viridans* is the most common cause of prosthetic valve endocarditis at other times; central venous catheters predispose to *Staphylococcus aureus* infection.
- *Intravenous drug misuse*: venepuncture without aseptic measures can introduce pathogens into the bloodstream, which may seed to the right side of the heart,

leading to tricuspid or pulmonary valve infection and incompetence. *Staphylococcus aureus* and *Candida albicans* are the main pathogens. *Staphylococcus aureus*, a skin commensal, causes an aggressive infection that leads to rapid, devastating damage to the heart and this is seen mainly in IV drug abusers.

Organisms implicated in IE

A summary of the main organisms causing IE is shown in Table 1.

Table 1 Common organisms and sources of infective endocarditis

Organism	Common sources
Streptococcus viridans (30–40% of all cases)	Upper respiratory tract
	Mouth
Enterococcus	Bowel
Other streptococci	Bowel, urine
Staphylococcus aureus	Skin
Staphylococcus epidermidis	Skin, prosthetic
Haemophilus	Upper respiratory tract
Anaerobes	Bowel
Fungi, e.g. *Candida*	Skin, bowel

Clinical features

Features of IE are often non-specific, including extreme tiredness and lethargy, loss of appetite and weight loss. Other features may include:

- *Results of infective emboli* – which may give rise to acute ischaemic ulcers, e.g. of the digits. These may be very painful, and may necessitate amputation.
- *Results of vasculitis:*
  - *splinter haemorrhages* – small, dark lines along the nail ridges
  - *clubbing of the nails* – a late phenomenon
  - *Osler's nodes* – painful nodules on the palmar aspect of the hands
  - *Roth spot* – a small, well-demarcated pale area of the fundus of the eye.
- *Splenomegaly.*
- *Cardiac consequences:*
  - *Heart murmur* – infection of a heart valve may lead to its damage, and the valve becoming incompetent, leading to a regurgitant murmur.
  - *Heart failure* – a consequence of valvular damage and subsequent incompetence. It is a serious finding in IE, since it signifies severe damage to the heart, and is an absolute indication for emergency valve replacement.

Investigations

Blood cultures

Blood cultures are vital. Multiple blood culture samples from multiple sites should ideally be taken before antibiotic therapy is given. Three sets of blood cultures have a sensitivity of over 90% in detection of the causal organism in IE.

Electrocardiography
ECG may show heart block (lengthening of the PR interval >0.2 second), indicating damage to the cardiac conduction tissue.

Chest radiograph
A chest radiograph may show signs of cardiac failure: cardiomegaly, pulmonary oedema, upper lobe diversion of blood. Cardiomegaly may also be a sign of valvular regurgitation caused by damage in IE.

Echocardiography
Echocardiography is used to assess valvular function and detect any vegetation or abscess. Transoesophageal echocardiography (TOE) has a higher sensitivity than transthoracic echocardiography; it can detect smaller vegetations and can be used to examine prosthetic valves. However, TOE is technically more difficult to perform. The absence of an echocardiographical evidence of IE does *not* exclude its presence.

Urine dipstix
A urine dipstix may reveal microscopic haematuria.

Other blood investigations
IE is associated with raised inflammatory markers such as erythrocyte sedimentation rate (ESR), C-reactive protein (CRP) and white blood cell (WBC) count.

Management

Medical
Empirical antibiotic treatment with intravenous (IV) benzylpenicillin plus IV gentamicin should be initiated immediately if IE is suspected, unless *Staphylococcus aureus* is suspected, when empirical therapy should be IV vancomycin plus IV gentamicin.

After identification of the causative organism with blood cultures, antibiotic therapy should then be focused on treatment of that organism.

Treatment for other commonly isolated organisms is shown in Table 2. The duration of antibiotic treatment is usually at least 2–4 weeks.

Table 2 Recommended antibiotic regimes for common causes of infective endocarditis

Organism	Antibiotic
Streptococcus (incl. *Enterococcus*)	IV benzylpenicillin /IV amoxicillin plus IV gentamicin
Staphylococcus sensitive to flucloxacillin	IV flucloxacillin plus IV gentamicin
MRSA/*Staphylococcus* resistant to flucloxacillin	IV vancomycin plus IV gentamicin

Surgical

Emergency surgical valve replacement should be considered in any patient with IE who is not responsive to antibiotic treatment, in patients with haemodynamic compromise (e.g. hypotension, heart failure) and in patients with a cardiac abscess.

Prevention of IE

Individuals with prosthetic heart valves or with congenital heart disease should take measures to prevent IE. Most importantly, there should be good oral hygiene and prompt treatment of any other source of infection, e.g. skin wounds.

Certain procedures are prone to the production of bacteraemia, and these should be covered with prophylactic antibiotics:

- Urological procedures should be covered with IV amoxicillin 1 g plus IV gentamicin 120 mg at induction. Amoxicillin 500 mg orally should be given 6 hours later. (Vancomycin should be used if allergic to penicillin.)
- Dental procedures under local anaesthetic should be covered with amoxicillin 3 g orally 1 hour before the procedure. (Clindamycin should be used if allergic to penicillin.)
- Dental procedures under general anaesthetic should be treated with IV amoxicillin 1 g at induction, plus amoxicillin 500 mg orally 6 hours later. (Vancomycin should be used if allergic to penicillin.)

Dental aspects

It is obligatory to try to prevent the onset of infective endocarditis in view of the high morbidity and mortality. Viridans streptococci are increased where oral hygiene is lacking, and can be released into the bloodstream in large numbers, particularly during tooth extractions or manipulations involving the periodontium.

Planned preventative oral health care is needed for all patients at risk of IE, such as those who have prosthetic heart valves or who have already had infective endocarditis, and those with congenital or rheumatic heart disease. Theoretically, antibiotics might be given for almost any dental procedure but, since both the necessity and efficacy of prophylaxis is unproven, the stage can be reached when the adverse effects from antimicrobials could outweigh any protection they might give.

Procedures needing antimicrobial prophylaxis in patients at risk of IE include:

1. extractions
2. subgingival procedures, including scaling
3. oral or periodontal surgery or raising mucogingival flaps for any other purpose (including implants).

Other suggested indications for antimicrobial prophylaxis, that may be of concern, but where the risks of antimicrobial prophylaxis may outweigh any theoretical benefits, include:

1. endodontic manipulation beyond the root apex
2. orthodontic banding
3. intraligamentary injections
4. incision or drainage of an abscess.

Procedures for which antimicrobial prophylaxis is *not* a requirement in persons at risk from IE include:

1. dental radiography
2. most endodontics
3. exfoliation of primary teeth
4. impression-taking
5. non-surgical procedures that do not induce bleeding
6. suture removal.

Five facts

1. Infective endocarditis (IE) is infection of the endocardium, especially the heart valves.
2. IE needs urgent medical treatment since it may lead to destruction of the heart valve, with subsequent heart failure.
3. The most common infection causing IE is *Streptococcus viridans*, which may spread from the oral cavity or upper respiratory tract.
4. IE can only be diagnosed with echocardiography.
5. Planned preventative oral health care is needed for patients with a prosthetic heart valve, previous IE, valvular, rheumatic or congenital heart disease, who are all at high risk for IE.

Inflammatory bowel disease

Inflammation of the colon is termed colitis, but there are several different types:

- ulcerative colitis (UC)
- Crohn's disease
- infective colitis (e.g. amoebic, *Campylobacter* or antibiotic-associated colitis – pseudomembranous colitis due to *Clostridium difficile*)
- ischaemic colitis due to mesenteric ischaemia (e.g. due to blockage of the artery by inadvertent ligation, embolus or atherosclerosis).

UC and Crohn's disease are collectively referred to as inflammatory bowel disease (IBD).

Ulcerative colitis

Ulcerative colitis is an inflammation of the rectum mainly, which can extend up the colon. The aetiology is uncertain but environmental factors, HLA B27 and autoimmunity appear to play a part. UC involves the mucosa with superficial ulceration, exudation and pseudopolyposis (ulcers with oedematous tags of mucosa between them). Because the bowel wall is oedematous and rigid, there is loss of the normal haustrations seen on X-ray. Even though there is inflammation of the bowel, it does not adhere to other intra-abdominal viscera, and thus fistulation is not a feature.

Clinical features
- Bloody diarrhoea and/or mucus per rectum (PR).
- Crampy abdominal pain.
- Tender left iliac fossa (LIF).
- Fever.
- Anorexia.
- Weight loss.

Investigations
Full blood count
Full blood count (FBC) will show microcytic anaemia due to blood loss.

Rigid sigmoidoscopy
Rigid sigmoidoscopy ('the siggy') shows mucosal granulation with contact bleeding and possibly pus. This can be an outpatient procedure, and biopsies can be taken for histological confirmation of the diagnosis.

Colonoscopy
Colonoscopy is useful to investigate the entire large bowel and determine the proximal extent of disease.

Barium enema
Barium enema may show oedema and fibrosis, with loss of haustrations, leading to a 'drainpipe colon'.

Differential diagnosis
- Crohn's disease.
- Infection.
- Colorectal cancer.

Because colorectal carcinoma more often presents with change in bowel habit compared to UC and Crohn's disease, which more commonly present with PR bleeding, most surgeons would opt for a colonoscopy for patients with change in bowel habit, and a barium enema for the PR bleeders. However, there is no hard and fast rule and these specialist investigations are the remit of the surgeon, not the dentist or GP.

Complications
Local complications
- Toxic megacolon – the bowel dilates hugely and is susceptible to perforation, a medical emergency that usually requires immediate surgical resection.
- Haemorrhage, leading to a microcytic anaemia.
- Stricture.
- Colorectal carcinoma develops in 15% of UC patients at 15 years, and thus patients should have 2-yearly colonoscopies and biopsies.

General complications ('extra-gastrointestinal manifestations')
- Anaemia.
- Weight loss.
- Arthritis.
- Rashes, e.g. pyoderma gangrenosum or erythema nodosum.
- Uveitis.
- Primary sclerosing cholangitis.
- Thromboembolic disease.

Management
Medical
- High protein diet with vitamin, iron and potassium supplements to replace electrolyte losses in the stools.
- Antidiarrhoeals.
- Anti-inflammatories.
- Corticosteroids in an acute attack.
- Salicylates to maintain remission.
- Psychological support.

Surgical
Surgical treatment is by resection of the involved segment of bowel. The extent of surgery depends on the extent of the UC, but typically it is either a colectomy with ileo-anal anastomosis, a permanent ileostomy or an ileo-anal pouch.

The indications for surgery are:

- severe disease unresponsive to medical management (such as >6 bloody motions per day with systemic illness)

- long-standing disease and risk of malignancy
- toxic megacolon
- stricture
- uncontrollable bleeding.

Crohn's disease

Crohn's disease is also sometimes referred to as 'terminal ileitis' or 'regional ileitis', as the terminal ileum is involved in >90% of cases. However, it can affect any part of the alimentary tract from mouth to anus (from 'top to tail') and, in rare instances, patients have presented with apparent appendicitis!

Clinical features

The clinical features of Crohn's disease are similar to UC and the distinction is often made on biopsy; however, Crohn's disease more commonly presents with anal fistulae and perianal abscesses, and in Crohn's disease the inflammation is throughout the bowel wall (transmural) – making bowel obstruction and malabsorption syndromes more likely.

Diagnosis

There is no specific diagnostic test for Crohn's disease.

- The ESR (erythrocyte sedimentation rate) and levels of other acute phase proteins such as C-reactive protein and seromucoid are usually raised.
- Serum potassium, zinc and albumin are usually depressed.
- Deficiencies of iron, folate or vitamin B_{12}, or anaemia may be found. The diagnosis of Crohn's disease is confirmed by sigmoidoscopy, colonoscopy and mucosal biopsy which often shows typical granulomas.
- Barium enemas of large and small bowel, or barium meal and follow-through may aid diagnosis.
- Ultrasound or isotope leukocyte intestinal scans may help to diagnose active disease.

Management

Treatment includes:

- sulfasalazine or newer 5-aminosalicylates (balsalazide, mesalazine or olsalazine)
- local corticosteroids
- surgery (usually resection) becomes necessary at some stage in most patients with intestinal Crohn's disease.

The management of Crohn's disease is more often medical, with surgery reserved for complications such as fistulation and abscesses, because Crohn's disease is discontinuous with affected areas of bowel sandwiched between normal areas (so-called skip lesions), making surgical resection difficult. This may explain why Crohn himself was a physician (at Mount Sinai Hospital, New York) rather than a surgeon!

Ulcerative colitis versus Crohn's disease

A comparison of UC with Crohn's disease is given in Table 1.

Table 1 Comparison of UC with Crohn's disease

	UC	*Crohn's disease*
Main sites affected	Rectum	Ileum
Disease distribution	Continuous from rectum	Discontinuous, anywhere from mouth to anus with skip lesions
Small bowel	Not affected	Typically affected
PR bleeding	Common	Less common
Perianal abscesses and fistulae	Rare	Common
Inflammation	Mucosal	Transmural
Pseudopolyps	Yes	No
Granulomas	No	Yes
Risk of malignant change	Moderate	Low
Surgery required	Commonly	Only for complications

Dental aspects

- Drugs that could aggravate inflammatory bowel disease should be avoided. These include non-steroidal anti-inflammatory drugs (NSAIDs), and antibiotics that could aggravate diarrhoea, e.g. amoxicillin–clavulanate and clindamycin.
- Oral lesions may be caused by the diseases or by associated nutritional defects. Oral ulceration may be seen in either UC (pyostomatitis vegetans) or Crohn's disease. Oral lesions of Crohn's disease include ulcers, facial or labial swelling, mucosal tags or 'cobblestone' proliferation of the mucosa. Oral effects of malabsorption such as angular stomatitis may also be seen. Some of these patients may have asymptomatic intestinal disease, or develop intestinal disease later.
- Orofacial granulomatosis (OFG) is the term given to granulomatous lesions similar to those of Crohn's disease, found on oral biopsy, but in the absence of detectable systemic disease. Melkersson–Rosenthal syndrome (facial swelling, facial palsy and fissured tongue) and cheilitis granulomatosa may also be incomplete manifestations of Crohn's disease.
- The finding of non-caseating granulomas beneath cobblestone proliferation of the oral mucosa is strongly suggestive of Crohn's disease or a variant.

Five facts

1. There are two main types of inflammatory bowel disease: ulcerative colitis (UC) and Crohn's disease.
2. Diarrhoea, PR bleeding and general systemic effects are common.
3. Extra-gastrointestinal manifestations include arthritis, uveitis, rashes and erythema nodosum.
4. UC (and to a lesser extent Crohn's disease) has a risk of malignant change after 10–15 years.
5. Oral ulceration is not uncommon in Crohn's disease and orofacial granulomatosis.

Ischaemic heart disease

Ischaemic heart disease (IHD, also known as coronary heart disease) results from inadequate blood supply to the myocardium via the coronary arteries. It includes a range of disorders from stable angina, to acute coronary syndrome, cardiac failure and arrhythmias.

Epidemiology

IHD is the main cause of death in the developed world. In the UK, approximately 25–30% of people die of IHD. Rates are slightly higher in men, high in Africans and Asians, and also rise with increasing age of the patient.

Clinical features

Stable angina
The typical features are exertional chest pain and shortness of breath. The pain is tight/heavy in the central chest (classically described as 'like an elephant sitting on my chest, doctor'), and with radiation to the neck and/or arms. The pain comes on over a few seconds and, after rest, it typically eases after a few minutes.

Acute coronary syndrome
The pain is identical to that in stable angina, except that it occurs at rest and persists for >15 min. In addition, the patient may feel short of breath, and may complain of nausea and vomiting.

Cardiac failure
Symptoms consist of shortness of breath, especially on exertion and when laying flat (orthopnoea). In addition, patients may complain of paroxysmal nocturnal dyspnoea (waking up gasping for breath).
   Signs include:

- raised JVP (jugulo-venous pressure)
- displacement of the apex beat
- bi-basal course crackles in the lungs (indicating pulmonary oedema)
- reduced air entry at the bases (indicating bilateral pleural effusions)
- pitting oedema in the legs.

Arrhythmias
The patient may complain of palpitations, near syncope (faintness) or even syncope (blackout). The pulse is irregular, and the patient may by hypotensive.

Risk factors for IHD

Smoking
The most important risk factor is *smoking*.

Other risk factors

- *Hypertension.*
- *Diabetes.*
- *Obesity.*
- *Hyperlipidaemia*: xanthomata (lipid deposits in tendons); xanthelasma (lipid deposits on the face); and corneal arcus. High blood cholesterol is one of the major risk factors for IHD. Dietary fat is processed by the liver to form four main lipoproteins: chylomicrons; very low density lipoproteins (VLDL); low density lipoproteins (LDL); and high density lipoproteins (HDL). VLDL reforms to LDL, and these fats are incorporated into atherosclerotic plaques, and associated with a high risk of IHD. By contrast, HDL clear cholesterol from the blood via the liver, appear to be anti-atherogenic, and are associated with a lower risk of IHD.
- *Family history* of IHD.
- *Homocysteinuria* is common but of controversial importance.

Pathology

Atherosclerosis (arteriosclerosis)

The overwhelming cause of ischaemic heart disease (and ischaemic stroke and peripheral vascular disease) is atherosclerosis – an inflammatory process which results in the formation of a plaque in the intima of an artery.

Plaque formation is initiated by the migration of monocytes from the blood into the intima to become macrophages. These macrophages engulf LDL cholesterol to become foam cells. Foam cells promote an inflammatory reaction by attracting smooth muscle cells, which change behaviour to make fibrous tissue. A plaque consisting of fibrous tissue, cholesterol and inflammatory cells therefore results and may self-propagate.

Stable angina

Angina is myocardial ischaemia caused by inadequate oxygen delivery for the heart demands. If the lumen of a coronary artery is narrowed due to atherosclerotic disease, the blood supply to that part of the myocardium will be deficient during exercise, when oxygen demand is increased, and there is anaerobic metabolism with the production of lactate and other acids, producing pain.

Acute coronary syndrome

Acute coronary syndrome (ACS) includes unstable angina and myocardial infarction (MI). Both syndromes are caused by coronary artery occlusion, which can occur in one of two ways:

1. the plaque surface ulcerates, and the resultant thrombus occludes the arterial lumen
2. the plaque progressively enlarges until it occludes the arterial lumen.

Unstable angina is ischaemia but no infarction. Myocardial infarction (a heart attack) is infarction of cardiac tissue as a result of interruption to its blood supply. Some MIs do not involve the full thickness of the myocardium, and so produce suggestive electrocardiogram (ECG) changes of unstable angina instead of an MI and are referred to as non-ST elevation myocardial infarctions (NSTEMIs).

Investigations

Electrocardiogram
ECG is a simple screening method for ischaemic heart disease. It may show changes such as evidence of ischaemia (ST depression, T-wave inversion), infarction (ST elevation, Q waves), hypertrophy of ventricles or arrhythmias.

Chest radiograph
A chest radiograph may show signs of cardiac failure, i.e. cardiomegaly, pulmonary oedema and/or bilateral pleural effusions.

Echocardiogram
An echocardiogram provides accurate information on heart function and structure and can therefore be used to detect and measure any heart failure.

Exercise tolerance test
An exercise tolerance test (treadmill test) is used to test for cardiac ischaemia on exertion. It is useful in stratifying the risk of patients with angina of future development of myocardial infarction. A high-risk patient would be investigated with coronary angiography.

Coronary angiography
Coronary angiography is the gold standard for diagnosing coronary artery disease. A catheter is inserted via the femoral artery to the coronary arteries in order to inject radiological contrast medium, which allows any stenosis or occlusion to be seen.

24-hour tape
A 24-hour ECG facilitates the identification of paroxysmal (intermittent) arrhythmias. It is performed in patients who give a history suggestive of an arrhythmia, but whose baseline ECG shows a normal (sinus) rhythm.

Cardiac enzymes
Troponin I/T are cardiac enzyme assays with 100% cardiac specificity. A raised troponin concentration indicates that an NSTEMI has occurred rather than unstable angina.

Screening
Screen for risk factors of atherosclerosis, e.g. serum lipids, fasting blood glucose and blood pressure (BP).

Management

Stable angina
Medical treatment includes the following:
- *Sublingual glyceryl trinitrate (GTN)* is used in acute pain to provide symptomatic relief. GTN acts to dilate the veins and arterioles, which reduces the preload and

afterload of the heart, respectively. Myocardial oxygen demand is therefore reduced. GTN also dilates coronary arteries, increasing myocardial perfusion. *Oral nitrates* are slow-release preparations of GTN, which provide a longer duration of action.

- *Beta-blockers* act on the heart to reduce its oxygen demand by reducing the rate and myocardial contractility. They also reduce blood pressure to further reduce the work done by the heart.
- *Calcium channel antagonists* reduce blood pressure via vasodilatation (mainly done by nifedipine and amlodipine) and reduce myocardial contractility (mainly done by verapamil).
- *Potassium channel activators*, e.g. nicorandil, act by causing arterial and venous dilatation.

If medical therapy provides poor control of angina, coronary angiography should be performed, and interventional treatment should be considered:

- *Percutaneous transluminal coronary angioplasty (PTCA)* is a radiological technique which involves the dilatation of a stenosed coronary artery using a balloon. Sometimes a stent is also placed across the stenosis to prevent early recurrence.
- *Coronary artery bypass graft (CABG) surgery*: in three-vessel disease, open surgery is used to graft either the saphenous vein or internal mammary artery to replace a section of each affected coronary artery.

Unstable angina/NSTEMI
Anyone with persistent (>15 min) chest pain, which sounds 'cardiac' in nature, should be managed as if they have unstable angina or an NSTEMI, even in the absence of positive ECG changes:

- *High-flow oxygen*
- *aspirin and clopidogrel* – to inhibit platelet function and coronary thrombus propagation
- *Intravenous GTN infusion* – to decrease myocardial oxygen demand and increase its blood supply
- *Beta-blocker* – to decrease the work of the heart
- *Low molecular weight heparin*, e.g. enoxaparin – to anticoagulate the patient.

Myocardial infarction
Anyone with persistent chest pain, with suggestive ECG changes of an MI or positive cardiac enzymes, should be treated as follows:

- *Thrombolysis* within 12 hours of onset of symptoms has been shown to substantially decrease mortality and morbidity and should be performed immediately, in patients with an ECG that confirms MI, using either streptokinase or tissue plasminogen activator. The most serious risk of thrombolysis is a 1% chance of haemorrhagic stroke. Other risks include hypotension and arrhythmias. Thrombolysis is absolutely contraindicated within 1 month of major surgery, with

any past history of cerebral haemorrhage or in uncontrolled hypertension. It is relatively contraindicated in pregnancy, proliferative diabetic retinopathy and recent trauma.
- PTCA (with or without stenting) is superior to thrombolysis in the acute treatment of MI, but its availability in the UK is still limited.

Other treatments which have been shown to decrease mortality and morbidity post-MI include:

- *Aspirin/clopidogrel*
- *Beta-blockers*
- *ACE (angiotensin-converting enzyme) inhibitors* (particularly beneficial in the presence of cardiac failure or diabetes).

Prevention of IHD

Preventative treatment for IHD is aimed primarily at the reduction of progression of atherosclerosis. This is achieved by reduction of risk factors for IHD with measures such as:

- *Reduction of cholesterol levels* by:
  - cutting down saturated fat and cholesterol in the diet
  - drugs to lower LDL cholesterol, e.g. (1) statins (pravastatin, simvastatin, etc.); (2) bile acid sequestrants (colesevelam) or resins (colestyramine, colestipol); (3) nicotinic acid-related drugs (nicotinic acid and acipimox); and (4) fibrates (clofibrate, fenofibrate, gemfibrozil).
- *Losing weight.*
- *Greater physical activity.*
- *Stopping cigarette smoking.*
- *Controlling hypertension.*
- *Good glycaemic control* (see chapter on diabetes mellitus).
- Taking a *diet* high in marine triglycerides (fish such as salmon, tuna and mackerel contain omega-3 fatty acids) and fruit and vegetables, moderate alcohol consumption and less salt.

Dental aspects

Stress, anxiety, exertion or pain can provoke angina; effective painless anaesthesia is essential. An aspirating syringe may be used since adrenaline (epinephrine) in the anaesthetic may get into the blood and may (theoretically) raise the blood pressure and precipitate arrhythmias.

Elective care should be deferred for >3 months for patients with myocardial infarction, recent onset angina or unstable angina with recent development of bundle branch block. In any case, it should be given in hospital.

Patients with IHD appear to have more severe dental caries and periodontal disease than the general population. Whether these infections bear any causative relationship to heart disease remains controversial.

Five facts

1. IHD is caused by inadequate blood supply to the myocardium.
2. Cardiac chest pain (ischaemia or infarction) is typically central, tight and heavy in nature, and it may radiate to the neck and/or arms.
3. Classical ECG changes are ST depression and/or T-wave inversion during angina, and ST elevation and/or abnormal Q waves during an MI.
4. If you suspect unstable angina or MI, give oxygen, aspirin 300 mg, GTN, do an ECG and call for urgent medical attention.
5. Elective dental care should be performed in hospital, and be deferred for >3 months for patients with MI, recent onset angina or unstable angina with recent development of bundle branch block.

Liver disease

Functions of the liver

The main functions of the liver are:

- The metabolism, breakdown and excretion of drugs and endogenous products such as ammonia, bilirubin and sex steroids. Bilirubin's ultimate destination is bile, which is made by the liver. Bilirubin is not water-soluble (unconjugated bilirubin) and needs a carrier (albumin) to be transported to the liver. In the liver, bilirubin is combined with glucuronic acid and converted into water-soluble conjugated bilirubin. Conjugated bilirubin enters the bile to be excreted in the faeces. Bile salts are needed for the absorption of fats and fat-soluble vitamins. Sex steroids, such as the masculinizing hormone testosterone and the feminizing hormone oestrogen, are inactivated.
- Production of many important substances, such as albumin, blood clotting factors II, VII, IX and X, transporter proteins, complement, cholesterol and bile components.
- Storage of substances such as glycogen, fat-soluble vitamins (vitamins A, D, E and K), folate, vitamin B_{12} and minerals such as copper and iron.
- Maintenance of body homeostasis by regulation of blood levels of substances such as cholesterol and glucose.

In liver disease, there can be disturbances in any or all of these processes.

Parenchymal liver disease

Parenchymal liver disease may present as one of a number of clinical syndromes, and is caused by a range of different pathologies.

Clinical syndromes of liver disease

Hepatitis
Hepatitis is inflammation of the liver. Hepatitis is often, but not always, caused by viruses. Features include jaundice (accumulation of bilirubin in the blood, the skin and sclera of the eyes), pruritus (itching from accumulation of bile salts), pain in the right upper quadrant of the abdomen, lethargy, loss of appetite and weight loss.

Cholestasis
Cholestasis is when bile excretion is impeded. This may be because of biliary obstruction (e.g. gallstones, primary sclerosing cholangitis, pancreatic cancer) or because of drugs. Features include jaundice as well as pruritus, pale stool and dark urine.

Chronic liver disease
Chronic liver disease is the syndrome produced by sustained hepatitis and the pathological process of cirrhosis. Identical symptoms to those of hepatitis may be present. In addition, characteristic signs such as clubbing, Dupuytren's contracture, palmar erythema, spider naevi, gynaecomastia, sialosis (salivary gland swelling) and hepatomegaly may be seen.

Patients may develop portal hypertension as a result of cirrhosis. This gives rise to features such as ascites (an abnormal accumulation of fluid in the peritoneal cavity), oesophageal varices and dilated abdominal veins in the skin (caput medusae). Varices are at high risk of life-threatening bleeding.

Liver failure
Liver failure may occur as a consequence of hepatitis, or as the end point of chronic liver disease. Clotting factors may be deficient, with resultant bleeding, and the reduced metabolism of toxins may lead to hepatic encephalopathy and hepatorenal syndrome (acute renal failure). Metabolic disturbances such as hypoglycaemia, hypocalcaemia and hypokalaemia may be present. The reduced blood albumin leads to oedema and hypotension. Cerebral oedema may occur, as well as increased susceptibility to infection.

Causes of parenchymal liver disease

Viruses

Hepatitis A
Hepatitis A (HAV) is an enterovirus transmitted via the faecal–oral route. With an incubation period of 2–4 weeks, it produces acute diarrhoeal illness or acute hepatitis. This only rarely leads to liver failure, and not to chronic liver disease. The Havrix inactivated vaccine is used to prevent HAV infection.

Hepatitis B
Hepatitis B (HBV) is a hepadnavirus. It may be transmitted by blood-borne spread (including blood transfusion and shared needles used by intravenous (IV) drug abusers), sexual contact or other bodily fluids such as saliva and urine. Several serological markers are associated with HBV infection or immunity, as shown in Table 1.

Table 1 Serological markers for hepatitis B

Serological markers for hepatitis B	Significance of presence of serological marker
HBsAg (surface antigen)	Current infection
HBeAg (e antigen)	Current infection associated with high infectivity
HBcAb (antibody to core antigen)	Infection in the present or past
HBsAb (antibody to surface antigen)	Immunity to HBV either via vaccination then also (HBcAb–ve) or past infection (HBcAb+ve)
HBeAg (antibody to e antigen)	Low infectivity

Most HBV infection results in acute hepatitis with complete and spontaneous resolution. However, in about 1% of cases the patient dies, in 5–10% of cases, infection may be chronic and, in about 20% of these, cirrhosis develops. The only effective treatment for chronic HBV is interferon. High-risk individuals such as dentists, doctors and nurses are routinely vaccinated using a recombinant HBsAg vaccine to prevent HBV infection.

Hepatitis C
Hepatitis C (HCV) is a flavivirus that accounts for the majority of transfusion-associated hepatitis. Blood-borne spread is by far its main route of transmission; however, sexual and vertical transmission may occur.

Most hepatitis C cases become chronic, with about 80% progressing to chronic liver disease, a proportion of whom develop liver cancer (hepatocellular carcinoma). A combination of interferon and ribavirin is used to treat chronic HCV. There is no vaccine yet to prevent HCV infection.

Hepatitis D
Hepatitis D (HDV) is an RNA virus which does not have the genetic code to replicate itself and therefore only infects hosts which are infected with HBV, whose replication proteins it uses to divide. HDV thus either coinfects hosts at the same time as HBV, or may superinfect hosts already chronically infected with HBV. HDV has the same modes of transmission as HBV.

Hepatitis D may lead to acute hepatitis, sometimes fulminating and lethal, or chronic liver disease. There is no vaccine to date.

Alcohol
Alcohol is metabolized in the liver and can damage it directly or via its breakdown products. Alcohol abuse is one of the main causes worldwide of chronic liver disease and cirrhosis. Currently, doctors suggest that men should drink less than 28 units a week, whereas women should drink no more than 21 units. A normal-sized glass of wine or half a pint of regular strength beer contains 1 unit. Regular drinking of small amounts of alcohol is thought to be safer than binge drinking to the same weekly amounts.

The key to management of alcoholic liver disease is the reduction or cessation of alcohol consumption, which should be supervised with specialist counselling.

Drugs
Drugs most noted for causing acute hepatitis include paracetamol (acetaminophen) in large doses, rifampicin and halothane. In most cases, cessation of the drug should lead to resolution of disease.

Paracetamol overdose is an important mode of suicide, since it can cause acute hepatitis and liver failure unless there is prompt treatment with *N*-acetylcysteine.

Halothane can produce an unusual allergic type of hepatitis, and repeated exposure should therefore be avoided.

Other causes
See Table 2 for other causes of parenchymal liver disease.

Neoplasms

Most liver neoplasms are metastases from primary tumours such as cancer of the lung, breast, bowel or pancreas.

The most common primary neoplasm of the liver is hepatocellular carcinoma (HCC), seen mainly in Asia and Africa. The main aetiological factors are cirrhosis (especially caused by HCV) and toxins such as aflatoxin (from a fungus infecting peanuts).

Table 2 Other causes of parenchymal liver disease

Main cause	Disease	Pathogenesis	Specific clinical features
Deposits	Haemo-chromatosis	A common disease of males, with overload of iron stores, leading to liver damage	Increased skin pigmentation Diabetes (bronze diabetes) Gonadal atrophy Cardiomyopathy
	Wilson's disease	Deficiency of biliary excretion of caeruloplasmin (containing copper)	Copper deposition in the basal ganglia causes extrapyramidal features Neuropsychiatric symptoms
Autoimmune	Primary biliary cirrhosis	Associated antibody: anti-mitochondrial	Classically affects middle-aged women Pruritus is the earliest feature
	Autoimmune hepatitis	Associated antibody: type I, anti-smooth muscle; type II, anti-LKM	Other autoimmune diseases, e.g. Hashimoto's thyroiditis, autoimmune haemolytic anaemia
Enzyme defect	α_1 anti-trypsin deficiency	Mutation in this serine protease inhibitor inhibits its excretion from the liver	Emphysema in early adulthood
Idiopathic	Primary sclerosing cholangitis	Leads to fibrosis of biliary tree, causing cholestasis	Association with ulcerative colitis, HIV

HCC may present with weight loss, tiredness, hepatomegaly, right upper quadrant pain, ascites or deranged liver function tests (LFT). The main methods of detection are a raised serum α-fetoprotein (AFP) or imaging with ultrasound or computed tomography (CT).

Curative surgery is possible in isolated lesions, but other patients need chemotherapy and/or embolization.

Thrombotic disease

The Budd–Chiari syndrome describes thrombotic obstruction of the hepatic veins or inferior vena cava. This leads to lack of venous drainage from the liver, which causes portal hypertension, acute hepatitis and even liver failure.

Liver abscesses/infective cysts

- *Pyogenic abscesses* may arise from cholangitis, haematological spread or from direct spread from abdominal infection.
- *Hydatid cysts* arise from infection with *Echinococcus granulosus*, a parasite found in some inadequately cooked lamb or goat meat seen mainly in the developing world.
- *Amoebic cysts* arise from gastrointestinal infection with the parasite *Entamoeba histolytica*, found in food or water contaminated with human faecal material mainly in the tropics.

The principle of management of all three conditions is aspiration of the lesion and antimicrobial or anti-protozoal therapy.

Investigations of liver disease

Liver function tests

Liver function tests are the simplest method of detecting hepatic dysfunction. A bilirubin concentration above 40 µmol/L may be detected clinically as jaundice and can be measured in the serum.

Liver serum enzymes

Alanine transaminase (ALT), aspartate transaminase (AST) and gamma-glutamyl transferase (γGT) are liver enzymes, increased serum levels of which usually indicate hepatitis; γGT is raised particularly where alcohol intake is high. Alkaline phosphatase (ALP), another liver enzyme, is raised in cholestasis.

Serum proteins
- *Serum albumin* is a good chronic marker of hepatic synthetic function.
- *Prothrombin time* is prolonged in hepatic failure, indicating deficient hepatic synthesis.
- *Serum caeruloplasmin* is measured to detect copper overload in Wilson's disease.
- *Serum α-fetoprotein*, if grossly raised, may indicate hepatocellular carcinoma.

Antibodies

Anti-mitochondrial antibodies are associated with primary biliary cirrhosis. Autoimmune hepatitis is associated with anti-smooth muscle and anti-LKM antibodies. Antibodies against HAV, HCV and HBV (see Table 1) are used to screen for viral hepatitis.

Serum iron studies

Serum iron studies are performed to assess for iron overload in haemochromatosis.

Ultrasound

Ultrasound of the liver is used to image the biliary tree for obstruction or, with CT, to image the liver to detect focal lesions (neoplasm or abscess/cyst) or diffuse changes such as fatty change or cirrhosis.

Liver biopsy

Liver biopsy provides the definitive diagnosis of parenchymal liver disease.

Management of liver disease

Chronic liver disease
Cessation/control of the underlying cause must be achieved wherever possible, e.g. cessation of alcohol intake. Complications such as liver failure and portal hypertension should be treated as below. Colestyramine may be used to reduce the pruritus produced by jaundice.

Portal hypertension
Portal hypertension may be treated in a number of ways.

1. Sodium and water restriction.
2. Diuretics: mainly spironolactone.
3. Paracentesis (drainage of ascites): may be needed periodically if ascites becomes tense and painful or affects breathing.
4. Shunts: Denver and LeVeen shunts deliver ascitic fluid from the peritoneum to the internal jugular vein and prevent backflow. TIPS (transjugular intrahepatic portosystemic shunting) is a radiological procedure used to place a stent between the portal vein and an hepatic vein, therefore reducing portal venous pressure.

Liver failure
Patients with acute liver failure should be treated in a high dependency or intensive care setting. Close observation and treatment of complications must be initiated:

- *Clotting factor deficiency:* vitamin K (necessary for hepatic production of clotting factors) and, if necessary, fresh frozen plasma (FFP), should be given according to the clotting profile of the patient.
- *Metabolic disturbances* such as hypoglycaemia, hypokalaemia and hypocalcaemia should be corrected.
- *Hepatic encephalopathy:* a low-protein diet is given to reduce nitrogen toxin production. Regular lactulose is given, which is metabolized by colonic bacteria, reduces the colonic pH and therefore reduces the ammonia produced by these bacteria. Neomycin is an antibiotic which is an alternative to lactulose where diarrhoea is a problem.
- *Hypotension*, which is monitored with central venous pressure (CVP) measurement, is treated with human albumin solution.
- *Liver transplantation*: any individual with liver failure should be considered for referral to a specialist liver unit for transplant assessment.

Dental aspects
- Disorders associated with a rise in serum levels of conjugated bilirubin in infants (e.g. biliary atresia) can cause a greenish discoloration of the developing teeth.
- Patients with parenchymal liver disease have impaired haemostasis and can present serious bleeding problems if oral surgery is needed.
- Impaired drug detoxification and excretion mean that the effects of many drugs are not entirely predictable.
- Local anaesthesia is safe in normal doses.

- Relative analgesia with nitrous oxide/oxygen is preferable to IV sedation with a benzodiazepine.
- Saliva and blood may contain hepatitis viruses.

Five facts

1. The most important functions of the liver are synthesis of substances such as albumin and clotting factors, and excretion of waste products and drugs.
2. Signs of chronic liver disease are jaundice, clubbing of fingers, palmar erythema, spider naevi, gynaecomastia and ascites.
3. The most important causes of chronic hepatitis are alcohol and viruses such as HBV and HCV.
4. People with liver failure have prolonged wound healing and deficient clotting.
5. Opioids (such as morphine), sodium intake (e.g. IV saline) and paracetamol (acetoaminophen) should be avoided in liver failure.

Lung cancer

Lung cancer (bronchial carcinoma) is the commonest malignant neoplasm affecting men in the developed world and is the commonest cause of death from cancer. Lung carcinoma is also the second commonest cancer in women after breast cancer, but is even more common than breast cancer in areas such as the West of Scotland where a high proportion of women smoke.

Cigarette smoking is the main cause of lung cancer. As more and more women are taking up smoking, the incidence of lung cancer in women is approaching that of men. Passive smoking, air pollution, asbestos exposure and radiation are other causative factors.

Clinical features

Commonly found features in patients suffering from bronchial carcinoma can be divided into features caused by tumour invasion and spread, and constitutional features.

Features caused by tumour invasion and spread
Recurrent chest infection
Recurrent pneumonia affecting the same lobe should raise suspicion of bronchial carcinoma.

Shortness of breath
Shortness of breath may either result from collapse/consolidation of a lung lobe by obstruction of its large airway(s) by tumour, or from a pleural effusion due to transcoelomic spread.

Haemoptysis
Haemoptysis (coughing of blood) occurs if the tumour invades a pulmonary blood vessel.

Chest pain
Chest pain is experienced from invasion of the pleura, chest wall or nerves.

Dysphagia
Dysphagia is caused by the tumour compressing the oesophagus.

Horner's syndrome
Horner's syndrome comprises miosis (constriction of the pupil), ptosis (drooping of the eyelid), anhidrosis (lack of sweat production) and enophthalmos on the affected side of the face. This arises from damage to the sympathetic nerve supply to the face by a bronchial carcinoma at the lung apex (often called a Pancoast's tumour).

Hoarseness
Hoarseness of voice occurs from tumour invasion of the left recurrent laryngeal nerve.

Superior vena caval obstruction
Superior vena caval (SVC) obstruction: bronchial carcinoma may spread via lymphatics to mediastinal and cervical lymph nodes, which can compress the SVC. This leads to engorgement of neck veins, a plethoric face and the formation of collateral vessels which are prominent on the upper praecordium (SVC syndrome).

Metastatic features
- Bone – bone pain, pathological fractures, anaemia.
- Liver – jaundice.
- Brain – seizures, neurological deficits, mood changes.

Constitutional features
Weight loss and malaise
Weight loss and malaise occur in patients suffering from bronchial carcinoma.

Clubbing of the fingers and toes
Clubbing consists of swelling of the tips of the digits, with loss of the nail-bed angle. Lung cancer is an important but not the solitary cause of clubbing.

Paraneoplastic syndromes
There are several paraneoplastic syndromes, most caused by hormone release from the tumour (ectopic hormone secretion), but all are rare.

Endocrine
Cushing's syndrome may arise from ectopic secretion of adrenocorticotrophic hormone (ACTH). Characteristic appearances including centripetal fat redistribution, proximal muscle wasting, moon facies and a buffalo hump.

Hypercalcaemia
Secretion of PTHRP (parathyroid hormone-related peptide) causes bone resorption and hypercalcaemia.

Syndrome of inappropriate antidiuretic hormone secretion (SIADH)
SIADH results in hyponatraemia, which may cause confusion, seizures or even coma.

Neurological
Lambert–Eaton syndrome is a myasthenia-like syndrome with muscle weakness and autonomic dysfunction. In contrast to myasthenia gravis, where there is weakness, sustained muscle contraction leads to an *increase* in muscle power.

Pathology

About half of lung cancers arise in the main bronchi, 75% being visible at bronchoscopy. The bronchial wall is narrowed and ulcerated and the cancer invades the lung parenchyma, and may cause necrosis, haemorrhage or abscess formation. If the cancer occludes the bronchus, the distal lung segments may collapse or become bronchiectatic.

The main types of lung cancer are:

- Squamous cell carcinomas (40%) – usually arise in an area of squamous metaplasia and are poorly differentiated. They often recur after resection, due to a 'field change' effect.
- Adenocarcinomas (30%) – usually are found in the periphery of the lung and grow rapidly. They cause an intense fibrotic (desmoplastic) response. These cancers are classically due to asbestos exposure rather than smoking.
- Large cell carcinomas (10%) – these are poorly differentiated and contain large cells with abundant cytoplasm.
- Small cell carcinomas (20%) – these comprise small cells with little cytoplasm, and produce peptides, giving rise to paraneoplastic syndromes (due to the remote effects of a hormone produced by the tumour). These tumours have a particularly poor prognosis, have generally spread even by the time of diagnosis, and are best treated with chemotherapy.

Other lung tumours include metastases from elsewhere, and carcinoid tumours. The latter are usually benign, but very occasionally can be malignant.

Metastases in the lung

The lung is a common site of metastasis from primary tumours in the breast (carcinoma), kidney (carcinoma), bone (sarcoma) and skin (melanoma). The classical coin-shaped lesion in the lung in a patient with renal cell carcinoma is termed a 'cannon ball' metastasis.

As lung metastases are so common, all patients with malignancy should have a chest radiograph.

Investigations

Investigations aim to establish the diagnosis, and to assess the stage (spread) and histological grade of the cancer in order to plan appropriate treatment.

Chest X-ray
A chest radiograph may show a mass in the lung field. Other features may include hilar lymphadenopathy (typically unilateral), collapse of a lung lobe or a pleural effusion on the side of the tumour.

Computed tomography
If suspicion of bronchial carcinoma is raised on a chest radiograph, a CT scan should be performed. This will show whether a mass seen on the plain film is likely to be a tumour. It will also show the extent of spread and lymphadenopathy.

Sputum cytology
Sputum cytology is a simple way to look for malignant cells but is not a substitute for biopsy.

Bronchoscopy

Bronchoscopy is performed to directly inspect the tumour and to obtain a tissue biopsy. If the tumour cannot be visualized on bronchoscopy, then CT-guided biopsy may be needed.

Management

In most cases the patient is incurable at the time of diagnosis. The overall 5-year survival rates are <25%. Surgical treatment consists of either removal of the affected lobe (lobectomy) or the whole lung (pneumonectomy), together with the affected lymph nodes. Non-surgical treatment consists of radiotherapy or chemotherapy. Radiotherapy may effectively treat non-resectable tumours if they have not metastasized. It is also useful for treatment of complications such as haemoptysis, or pain from chest wall invasion.

Chemotherapy is most useful for treating small cell carcinomas, and for non-resectable disease. One regime consists of cyclophosphamide, doxorubicin and vincristine.

Dental aspects

- Oral cancer may be associated with bronchial carcinoma, and vice versa, or develop at a later stage. Such *synchronous* or *metachronous* primary tumours must always be ruled out. Metastases can occasionally cause enlargement of the lower cervical lymph nodes or involve the jaw.
- Dental treatment under local anaesthesia should be uncomplicated. Conscious sedation should preferably be avoided.
- Lung cancer is a fairly common cause of death in dental technicians but this may be due as much to smoking as to dust inhalation.

Five facts

1. Lung cancer is the commonest cancer in men and the second commonest cancer in women in the UK.
2. Smoking is the main risk factor.
3. Passive smoking more than doubles the risk of developing lung cancer.
4. Lung cancer often presents late when it is inoperable.
5. Lung cancer can metastasize to the jaw.

Meningitis

The meninges, the membranes which surround the brain and spinal cord, consist of three layers:

- the *dura mater* is the outermost layer and is adherent to the skull
- the *arachnoid mater* is the middle layer
- the *pia mater* is the innermost layer and is adherent to nervous tissue

Cerebrospinal fluid (CSF) circulates in the space between the arachnoid and the pia (subarachnoid space).

Meningitis is inflammation of the meninges, usually caused by viral infection, but bacterial meningitis is the most deadly form.

Epidemiology

Meningitis can affect people of any age. Bacterial meningitis is a concern particularly in younger people, where it may occur in small epidemics in the community, transmitted by respiratory and direct spread.

Aetiology

Spread of microorganisms to the meninges is usually via the bloodstream.

Viral meningitis

Eighty per cent of cases of meningitis are viral; the majority of cases do not result in overt clinical meningitis, but rather cause a non-specific febrile illness which resolves spontaneously over a few days.

The enteroviruses (such as Coxsackie, polio, ECHO) account for most cases. Other viruses causing meningitis include influenza, mumps, herpes simplex, varicella zoster and HIV.

Bacterial meningitis

The causes of bacterial meningitis are classified according to the age group of the patient (Table 1).

Table 1 Classification of causes of bacterial meningitis by age of patient

Age of patient	Common causes	Less common causes
Neonate	Streptococcus group B	Listeria monocytogenes
Infant	Haemophilus influenzae	Neisseria meningitidis
		Streptococcus pneumoniae
Adult	Neisseria meningitidis	Streptococcus pneumoniae
		Haemophilus influenzae
Older person	Streptococcus pneumoniae	Neisseria meningitidis

Neisseria meningitidis (meningococcus types A, B and C) is the most common and dangerous cause of bacterial meningitis in the UK. Meningococcal meningitis is transmitted by respiratory and direct spread. A significant proportion of the population carry the bacterium in their nasopharynx but only rarely does bacterial meningitis result from such carriage. The reasons for this are unclear. Meningococcal meningitis is associated with meningococcal septicaemia, which may cause rapidly worsening shock and multi-organ failure.

Haemophilus influenzae and *Streptococcus pneumoniae* (pneumococcus) meningitis are sometimes associated with otitis media (infection of the middle ear). Pneumococcal meningitis may be associated with pneumonia.

Meningitis in the immunocompromised patient

Immunosuppression, e.g. due to HIV, lymphoma or chemotherapy, predisposes to all infections, including meningitis.

Meningitis may be caused by the usual pathogens (see above) plus opportunistic organisms such as *Mycobacterium tuberculosis* (which tends to cause chronic meningitis and may cause hydrocephalus), fungi (e.g. *Cryptococcus*) and protozoa (e.g. *Toxoplasma*).

Non-infectious meningitis

Neoplasms such as lymphoma and metastatic carcinoma (e.g. breast, lung) may deposit in the meninges and cause chronic meningitis. Inflammatory diseases such as systemic lupus erythematosus (SLE), sarcoidosis and Behçet's disease may all cause chronic meningitis.

Clinical features

All types of meningitis cause fever and meningeal irritation and thus the clinical syndrome of meningism – headache (classically a severe occipital headache), neck stiffness, nausea and vomiting.

The patient may be drowsy due to raised intracranial pressure associated with cerebral oedema and this can be fatal. Two neurological signs in particular may be positive:

- Kernig's sign: with the hip flexed, passive extension at the knee causes spasm in the thigh.
- Brudzinski's sign: passive flexion of the neck leads to involuntary hip flexion.

If the cause of meningitis is meningococcal, septicaemia with characteristic purpuric skin lesions may be evident.

Complications

Focal neurological deficit

The cerebral oedema causes the brain to swell and this may stretch cranial nerves and cause palsies, such as of the ophthalmic nerve (CN III), which runs from the brainstem and through the superior orbital fissure. These palsies are referred to as *false localizing signs* since they incorrectly imply that a focal lesion has affected function of a cranial nerve, rather than the diffuse process of meningitis. Note that any other cause of raised intracranial pressure such as a cerebral haemorrhage may also cause false localizing signs.

Hydrocephalus
Meningitis (especially caused by TB) may damage the arachnoid granulations and impair reabsorption of CSF. Excess CSF leads to dilatation of the brain ventricles, and subsequent hydrocephalus. Hydrocephalus causes drowsiness and cognitive impairment.

Seizures
Meningitis may irritate the parenchyma of the brain and cause seizures.

Coning
If cerebral oedema continues to progress, the brain may begin to herniate through the foramen magnum. If the medial parts of the temporal lobes squeeze through as well, they can compress the brainstem, causing dysfunction of cardiovascular and respiratory centres and death.

Investigations

Blood cultures
Blood cultures should be taken ideally before treatment but should *never* delay the administration of antibiotics.

Blood investigations
A raised white cell/neutrophil count and C-reactive protein (CRP) are consistent with infection. Serial measurement is useful to monitor response to therapy. Renal function should be monitored, since sepsis can cause renal failure.

Computed tomography
It is important to perform a CT scan of the head urgently in anyone presenting with impairment of consciousness and/or focal neurological deficit (e.g. a cranial nerve palsy). The first reason for this is that both features suggest the possibility of a focal lesion in the brain, e.g. tumour or subarachnoid haemorrhage. Diagnosis of which lesion is present obviously affects management. The second reason for doing an urgent CT is that lumbar puncture is absolutely contraindicated in the presence of a focal cerebral lesion. This is because removal of CSF from around the spinal cord would increase any pressure gradient in the CSF from the brain to the spinal cord, and therefore promote coning.

Lumbar puncture
Removal of a small volume of CSF is vital in the diagnosis of meningitis, and in identification of the causative agent. CSF should be sent for the following tests.

Microscopy
A raised CSF white cell count is in itself diagnostic of meningitis, whatever the cause (Table 2). A Gram stain should identify most bacteria. An auramine stain should be performed if TB is suspected. An Indian ink stain will detect *Cryptococcus neoformans*.

Culture of bacterial organisms
A special TB culture (Löwenstein–Jensen) may be set up if requested.

Biochemistry
Protein may be raised, and glucose may be low (see Table 2).

Table 2 Comparison of cerebrospinal fluid analysis for different causes of meningitis and a normal individual

CSF measurement	Normal	Bacterial meningitis	Viral meningitis	TB meningitis
White cell count	<5	500–5000 mm^3 neutrophils	50–1000 mm^3 lymphocytes	50–5000 mm^3 lymphocytes
Protein	Up to 0.5 g/L	High	Normal	High
Glucose	>2/3 serum glucose	Low	Normal	Low

Management

IT IS VITAL THAT EMPIRICAL ANTIBIOTICS ARE GIVEN IMMEDIATELY IF MENINGITIS IS SUSPECTED.

Under no circumstance should any investigation or result delay antibiotic treatment, since bacterial meningitis can progress and worsen over hours to be fatal.

Antibiotics
Empirical antibiotic therapy is high-dose intravenous (IV) cefotaxime (2 g four times a day) or ceftriaxone (2 g twice daily). However, if the patient has a typical rash of meningococcal septicaemia, high-dose IV benzylpenicillin (2.4 g four times a day) should be given instead.

If the causative organism is identified, antibiotic choice should be rationalized in order to specifically treat it. Meningococcus should be treated with benzylpenicillin, as described above. Pneumococcus or *H. influenzae* should be treated with cefotaxime or ceftriaxone.

Microbiological advice should be sought on antibiotic choice, particularly once sensitivity tests to antibiotics have been performed.

Other treatment
IV fluids and other supportive measures may be needed to treat sepsis and its complications. Seizures should be treated with diazepam and phenytoin (see chapter on epilepsy).

Immunization
A vaccine for Group B meningococcus, which accounts for the majority of cases, is not available. A vaccine for Group C meningococcus is available and all school children are now vaccinated; it is hoped that such vaccination will reduce the total incidence of meningococcal meningitis. Immunization is also available against some *H. influenzae* strains.

Contact tracing

All household and other close contacts of meningococcal meningitis should be treated with antibiotics to eradicate nasopharyngeal carriage. This is achieved with a single dose of ciprofloxacin, or with a short course of rifampicin.

Dental aspects

Spread of bacteria to the meninges is occasionally as a result of a maxillofacial fracture involving the cribriform plate of the ethmoid. Patients with maxillofacial injuries involving the middle third of the face should be given prophylactic antimicrobials because of the danger of meningitis.

Five facts

1. Meningitis is inflammation of the meninges, which is caused by infection (or rarely by non-infectious causes).
2. Most cases of meningitis are viral (80%).
3. The most common cause of bacterial meningitis is meningococcus (*Neisseria meningitidis*).
4. Empirical antibiotics must be given immediately if meningitis is suspected.
5. Patients with maxillofacial injuries involving the middle third of the face should be given prophylactic antimicrobials because of the danger of meningitis.

Neck swellings

The majority of surgical conditions that appear in the neck arise as a swelling.

Cervical lymphadenopathy

The commonest cause of a swelling in the neck is enlargement of a lymph node. Even if only one node is clinically palpable, adjacent non-palpable nodes are often also affected.
The main causes of cervical lymphadenopathy are:

- Infections: usually tonsillitis, glandular fever or upper respiratory tract infections (URTI), mouth infections and occasionally HIV, toxoplasmosis, syphilis or tuberculosis.
- Malignant disease: metastases (from primary tumours in the head and neck, chest or abdomen) and primary reticuloses (e.g. lymphoma, leukaemia).
- Sarcoidosis.

Tonsillitis

Tonsillitis is overall the commonest cause of cervical lymphadenopathy. Typically, the patient is a child complaining of a painful lump and a sore throat. More than four episodes of tonsillitis per year or a total of 13 attacks are indications for tonsillectomy. An infrequent complication of tonsillitis is peritonsillar abscess (quinsy), which can obstruct the airway and requires immediate surgical drainage followed later by tonsillectomy.

HIV

Cervical lymphadenopathy, as part of persistent generalized lymphadenopathy (PGL), is common in HIV/AIDS.

Tuberculosis

The tubercle bacillus (*Mycobacterium tuberculosis* or *M. bovis*) can enter the body via unpasteurized milk or inhalation, and via the tonsils can then enter the cervical lymph nodes, most commonly those of the deep cervical chain. The lump in the neck feels matted and can be painful. Increasing size of the swelling and pain plus overlying skin discoloration suggest the development of a tuberculous abscess. Such abscesses can burst through the deep fascia of the neck and become 'dumbbell' shaped. The skin temperature over tuberculous abscesses is normal because the process of caseation and pus formation is slow and does not stimulate excessive hyperaemia, and hence they are also termed 'cold' abscesses. When there are several cervical abscesses, the term 'scrofula' may be used. Non-tuberculous mycobacteria may present similarly.

Malignant disease

Malignant disease is the commonest cause of cervical lymphadenopathy in middle-aged or elderly adults. The nodes are non-tender and hard, classically 'stony' hard, to palpation. The primary cancer is most often in the oral cavity (tongue, lips and other mucous membranes) and larynx, but the entire drainage area of the cervical lymph nodes (head including face, neck, chest including breasts, and abdomen) must be thoroughly examined for a primary neoplasm. Full dental and ear, nose and throat (ENT) examinations are therefore vital. Occasionally, an enlarged cervical node is found in the absence of a detectable primary tumour. In those cases, biopsy of the tonsils and nasopharynx is indicated, since hidden primaries may be revealed.

The commonest of the primary neoplasms of lymph nodes (lymphoreticular disease) are leukaemia and malignant lymphomas, all potentially lethal. The acute leukaemias are seen mainly in children and are characterized by primitive blast cells in the blood and bone marrow. Chronic leukaemias are characterized by an excess of mature leukocytes in blood and bone marrow and are mainly diseases of adult life which are chronic disorders but may progress to acute leukaemia.

Many of the manifestations of leukaemia arise from the crowding out of normal blood cells from the marrow by the leukaemic cells, leading to anaemia (fatigue, pallor, etc.), thrombocytopenia (purpura and a bleeding tendency) and a liability to infections.

Lymphomas are seen mainly in young adults and are commonly divided into Hodgkin's disease and the more common non-Hodgkin's lymphoma. Typically, patients present with a painless, rubbery, posterior triangle neck lump, as well as the so-called 'B' symptoms of malaise, weight loss, pallor and swinging fevers (Pel–Ebstein fever). Some patients suffer from abdominal pain after drinking alcohol, although the mechanism for this is not understood. Other groups of lymph nodes may be enlarged, and patients with lymphoreticular disease should be examined for hepatosplenomegaly, anaemia and jaundice, and be referred to a haematologist. Staging is based on history, physical examination and investigations such as blood tests, biopsies (e.g. of lesions, lymph nodes and bone marrow) and imaging – radiography, computed tomography (CT) and magnetic resonance imaging (MRI) scans or ultrasound.

Treatment can be with surgery, radiotherapy, cytotoxic drugs singly or in combination, stem cell transplantation, immunotherapy (monoclonal antibodies and – on the horizon – vaccines) and gene therapy.

Branchial cyst

A branchial cyst is a remnant of a branchial cleft. Embryologically, there are six branchial clefts, and it is usually the second cleft that persists to form a branchial cyst. Hence, these cysts are lined with squamous epithelium, but there are also patches of lymphoid tissue in their walls which are connected with other lymph tissue in the neck and can become infected.

Most cysts present in the 15–25 age group as a painless swelling beneath the upper third of the sternocleidomastoid (SCM) muscle. The lump can become painful and increase in size when the lymph tissue in the cyst wall gets infected. The local deep cervical nodes should not be enlarged (if they are you should consider tuberculous abscess instead of branchial cyst as your diagnosis). Branchial cysts have no systemic effects and are not associated with any other congenital abnormality. They are commonly treated conservatively or by surgical excision.

Branchial fistula and sinus

A fistula is an abnormal communication between two epithelial surfaces. A branchial fistula is the remnant of a branchial cleft, usually the second, which has not closed off. The patient therefore presents with a small dimple at the junction of the middle and lower thirds of SCM that discharges clear mucus, and sometimes becomes swollen and discharges pus.

A sinus is a blind-ending track from an epithelial surface. In many cases of branchial 'fistula' the remnant of the branchial cleft opens onto the skin overlying the neck but is obliterated on the inside where it would embryologically connect with the oropharynx behind the tonsil. Hence, in these cases, the branchial 'fistula' is really a branchial sinus.

Branchial fistulae and sinuses are usually treated by surgical excision.

Chemodectoma

Also called a 'carotid body tumour', a chemodectoma is a rare, usually benign although occasionally malignant, tumour of the chemoreceptor tissue in the carotid body. Hence it lies at the carotid bifurcation, typically level with the hyoid bone, and beneath the anterior edge of SCM. Its distinguishing feature is that it pulsates. The patient may suffer from transient cerebral ischaemia (blackouts, transient paralysis or paraesthesiae) or palsies of the VII, IX, X, XI and XII cranial nerves (dysphagia, hoarseness), but this is unusual as the tumours are usually slow growing.

Duplex ultrasound, carotid angiography and MRI or CT scanning are often needed to determine the precise localization of the chemodectoma and its relation to the carotid and its bifurcation. It is vital for the vascular surgeon to have this information before attempting surgical removal.

Cystic hygroma

A cystic hygroma is a collection of lymphatic sacs which contain clear colourless lymph and is therefore also termed a lymphangioma. Cystic hygromas usually present at birth or infancy as fluctuant, transilluminable swelling in the base of the neck. They are usually managed by conservative means or surgical excision after localization with MRI to determine the relation of the hygroma to nearby vessels and nerves.

Pharyngeal pouch

This is a pulsion diverticulum of the pharynx through the gap between the lowermost horizontal fibres (cricopharyngeus) and the higher oblique fibres (thyropharyngeus) of the inferior constrictor muscle. With uncoordinated swallowing the sphincter-like cricopharyngeus fibres do not relax and cause the unsupported area just above these fibres (Killian's dehiscence) to bulge out. Eventually, the bulge grows into a sac which hangs down and presses against the side of the oesophagus.

Pharyngeal pouches typically occur in middle-aged and elderly men and present with halitosis, recurrent sore throats or regurgitation of food. Regurgitation at night causes bouts of coughing and choking, and if pieces of food are inhaled a lung abscess may develop. As the pouch grows, it may form a lump behind SCM (although commonly no lump is seen or felt), and it can compress the oesophagus and cause dysphagia.

Diagnosis is confirmed by a barium swallow, which shows contrast going down the diverticulum separate from the pharynx–oesophagus, and treatment is traditionally by excision of the pouch combined with a posterior cricopharyngeal myotomy, although endoscopic stapling of the pouch is becoming more common.

Sternocleidomastoid 'tumour'

A sternocleidomastoid 'tumour' is not a real tumour but an ischaemic contracture of a segment of SCM, classically the middle third. The ischaemia is caused by the trauma of birth and the baby presents with torticollis. Remember that contracture of the left SCM turns the head towards the right, but tilts it to the left, and vice versa. Patients with SCM tumours should be referred to a paediatric surgeon to confirm the diagnosis and advise whether conservative or surgical treatment is needed.

Cervical rib

The cervical rib is usually a fibrous band, although sometimes a fully developed rib, attached to the first cervical vertebra, and occurs in less than 1% of the population. It is bilateral in 50% of cases. Examination of the neck is usually normal although occasionally a fullness at the root of the neck can be felt. The importance of this condition is that it can cause serious neurological and vascular symptoms, typically pain and wasting in the C8 and T1 dermatomes, wasting and weakness of the small muscles of the hand, Raynaud's phenomenon, trophic changes and even gangrene of the hand. These symptoms are due to the compressive effects of the cervical rib and are indications for surgical removal by a vascular surgeon.

Thyroglossal cyst and fistula

The thyroid gland develops as a bud from the floor of the pharynx and descends through the tongue, past the hyoid, to its position in the neck. If a portion of its track remains patent, it can form a thyroglossal cyst. Hence these cysts occur in the midline anywhere along the line of thyroid descent (from the foramen caecum at the tongue base down to the thyroid isthmus) and are attached to the hyoid bone (as the track passes through this). As the track is attached to the tongue base, the cyst will ascend when the patient sticks his tongue out or swallows. Occasionally, the track will open out onto the surface of the neck and discharge fluid. This is a thyroglossal fistula and can become infected.

The management of thyroglossal cysts and fistulae is surgical excision. It is important to remove not just the cyst but also the entire track right up to the region of the foramen caecum, as well as the body of the hyoid that the track runs through (Sistrunk's operation). If this is not done, then the cyst/fistula can recur.

The thyroid gland itself can cause neck lumps and these are discussed in the chapter on thyroid disorders.

Dental aspects

Dentists should always include examination of cervical lymph nodes in their examination of patients, as oral pathology can present with cervical lymphadenopathy.

Five facts

1. Lymphadenopathy is the commonest cause of neck swelling.
2. Infections and malignancy are causes of enlarged cervical lymph nodes.
3. A midline neck swelling is most commonly of thyroid origin.
4. A swelling in the substance of the thyroid gland moves up on swallowing; a thyroglossal cyst moves up on tongue protrusion.
5. Oral pathology can cause cervical lymphadenopathy.

Nerve injuries

Nerve injuries may result from laceration (cutting), stretching (traction) or compression (crush) and, depending on the severity, may recover to varying extents.

There are three types of nerve injury:

1. *Neuropraxia* is damage to the nerve fibres but with no loss of contiguity to the surrounding axis cylinder. It may occur from prolonged pressure or friction. An example is a palsy of the common peroneal nerve from a tightly applied plaster cast. Neuropraxia is a 'concussion'-type injury and recovery begins within a few days and is usually complete in a few weeks.
2. *Axonotmesis* is injury to both the axon and its myelin sheath, without disruption of the surrounding perineural sheath. It causes the axon distal to the lesion to degenerate (Wallerian degeneration), but a new axon grows from the proximal node of Ranvier and, since the perineural sheath is intact, the correct axon will grow into the correct sheath. Nerve regrowth typically occurs at about 1 mm/day.
3. *Neurotmesis* is total disruption at a specific place. It leaves no sheath available to direct regrowth, which therefore depends on how close the two damaged nerve ends are. As perineural sheaths and axons regenerate independently and there is nothing to direct the correct axons into the correct sheaths, the result is a mismatch of new sprouting axons and sheaths. Hence, the patient may be left with a permanent disability, which rehabilitation may only partly resolve.

Neuropraxia and axonotmesis are usually diagnosed on clinical suspicion from partial impairment in function immediately after injury. The treatment is to splint in their position of function the joints whose muscles have been paralysed, so that contractures are avoided. Passive movements to maintain muscle bulk are important to allow function when the nerve injury resolves. The damaged nerve is itself not interfered with.

Neurotmesis presents with complete loss of function in the acute phase, and diagnosis is often confirmed at operative exploration. Such nerve injuries require early operative repair with careful apposition of the divided nerve ends but, if the ends are too far apart to appose without tension, nerve grafts or tendon transfers may be used.

Common individual nerve injuries

Common individual nerve injuries are listed in Table 1.

Brachial plexus injuries

Erb's palsy
Erb's palsy results from a lesion to the upper trunk of the brachial plexus and hence involves roots C5 and C6. The upper trunk is pulled out when the head is forced away from the shoulders, as occurs commonly in motorcycle accidents or after forceps obstetric deliveries. The limb assumes a 'waiter's tip' position – internal rotation with pronation (paralysis of brachioradialis, supinator and biceps brachii). The arm cannot be lifted or flexed (paralysis of deltoid, biceps and brachialis). Sensory loss affects

Table 1 Common individual nerve injuries

Nerve lesion	Causes	Classical motor loss	Classical sensory loss
Radial nerve	Fracture of humerus in spiral groove; Saturday night palsy after falling asleep drunk, with arm overhanging chair	Wrist drop (paralysis of wrist extensors) and inability to extend elbow (paralysis of triceps)	Over anatomical snuffbox (small area on dorsum of hand between thumb and index finger)
Median nerve	Fractures of elbow; laceration of forearm/wrist (e.g. deliberate self-harm as in a suicide attempt; carpal tunnel syndrome)	Paralysis of small muscles of thenar eminence with wasting; inability to abduct thumb; ulnar deviation of wrist on flexion	Over radial three and a half fingers on palmar surface
Ulnar nerve	Fractures of elbow; laceration of forearm/wrist; compression in Guyon's canal	All non-median supplied intrinsic hand muscles are paralysed, leading to inability to adduct and abduct fingers and wasting of the web spaces; claw hand deformity	Over ulnar one and a half fingers on palmar surface
Common peroneal nerve	Compression of neck of fibula in operating theatre or from a tight cast; bumper injury to pedestrian in road traffic accident	Inversion of foot and foot drop due to paralysis of peronei	Over anterior surface of foot and leg

the 'regimental badge' area over the upper arm (loss of the roots that supply the axillary nerve). The biceps and supinator reflexes will be absent.

Klumpke's palsy

Klumpke's palsy results from a lesion to the lowermost root of the brachial plexus, i.e. T1, most often due to a compression from a cervical rib or from a stretching injury separating the arm from the body (e.g. holding on to the edge of a wall or building to avoid falling). The T1 lesion leads to wasting of the small muscles of the hands (the interossei and lumbricals), and loss of sensation on the inner side of the forearm and ulnar three and a half fingers. If the sympathetic fibres from T1 are also affected, then Horner's syndrome (loss of sweating, miosis and ptosis) also results on the affected side.

Table 2 Cranial nerves, main lesions and features

Cranial nerve	Main features of lesions	Main causes
I	Anosmia or hyposmia	Trauma Infection Neoplasm
II	Visual defect or blindness	Trauma Infection Neoplasm Cerebrovascular accident Multiple sclerosis
III	Ptosis Dilated pupil	Diabetes Trauma
IV	Diplopia	Trauma
V	Anaesthesia or hypoaesthesia	Trauma Infection Neoplasm Multiple sclerosis Connective tissue disease
VI	Diplopia	Trauma Neoplasm Cerebrovascular accident Raised intracranial pressure
VII	Facial palsy	Trauma Infection Neoplasm Cerebrovascular accident Multiple sclerosis
VIII	Impaired hearing or deafness	Trauma Infection Neoplasm Cerebrovascular accident Bone disease
IX	Impaired gag reflex	Trauma Neoplasm
X	Impaired gag reflex Voice changes	Trauma Neoplasm Cerebrovascular accident
XI	Weakness on shrugging shoulders	Cerebrovascular accident Infection (polio)
XII	Tongue deviation and sometimes wasting	Trauma Neoplasm

Cranial nerve lesions with dental relevance

The cranial nerves most commonly damaged or diseased are the trigeminal and facial nerves (Table 2).

Damage to a sensory branch of the trigeminal nerve causes hypoaesthesia in its area of distribution, initially a diminishing response to pinprick to the skin and, later, complete anaesthesia.

Extracranial causes of facial sensory loss are most common and include damage to the trigeminal nerve from trauma – the usual cause – especially by inferior alveolar local analgesic injections, fractures or surgery (particularly surgical extraction of lower third molars, osteotomies or jaw resections), especially after orthognathic or cancer surgery. Uncommon causes include bone disease, malignant disease and neuropathies. Intracranial lesions are uncommon but serious and include:

- Inflammatory disorders:
  - disseminated (multiple) sclerosis
  - sarcoidosis
  - infections (e.g. HIV)
  - connective tissue disorders.
- Brain tumours.
- Syringobulbia.
- Drugs.

Table 3 Localization of site of lesion in, and causes of, unilateral facial palsy

Muscles paralysed	Probable site of lesion	Type of lesion
Lower face	Upper motor neurone (UMN)	Stroke
		Brain tumour
		Trauma
		HIV infection
All facial muscles	Lower motor neurone (LMN) Facial nucleus	Multiple sclerosis
All facial muscles	Between nucleus and geniculate ganglion	Fractured base of skull
		Posterior cranial fossa tumours
		Sarcoidosis
All facial muscles	Between geniculate ganglion and stylomastoid canal	Otitis media
		Cholesteatoma
		Mastoiditis
All facial muscles	In stylomastoid canal or extracranially	Bell's palsy (mostly HSV)
		Trauma
		Local analgesia (e.g. misplaced inferior dental block)
		Parotid tumour
		Other infections (e.g. Lyme disease)
Isolated facial muscles	Branch of facial nerve extracranially	Trauma
		Local analgesia

Facial palsy can follow stroke, or can be due to a lower motor neurone lesion. Bell's palsy may be immunologically mediated and most idiopathic cases are probably due to infection with herpes simplex virus (HSV). Facial palsy may be seen after other infections (e.g. HIV, VZV, CMV, EBV, influenza, HTLV-1, HIV and Lyme disease), or from trauma or tumours.

Trigeminal neuralgia is a lancinating severe pain which, though often idiopathic, may be caused by multiple sclerosis or brain tumour.

Five facts

1. Nerve injuries can be due to compression, laceration or traction.
2. Total disruption of the nerve (neurotmesis) usually results in permanent disability with only a partial recovery.
3. Bell's palsy leads to facial muscle weakness on the side of the lesion.
4. Brain tumours and space-occupying lesions within the skull can lead to a variety of cranial nerve palsies.
5. The facial nerve may be injured by a facial laceration or stab.

Pain and analgesia

Physiology of pain

In order to treat pain, it is important to have a basic appreciation of the structure and function of the pathways involved in the transmission of painful stimuli:

1. Painful stimuli activate pain receptors (free nerve endings of peripheral afferent nociceptors).
2. Nociceptors may be small and myelinated (A-*delta* fibres; for the transmission of 'fast' pain), or large and unmyelinated (C fibres; for conveying chronic pain).
3. The afferent nerve fibres convey the impulse to the spinal cord dorsal horn of the grey matter, and synapse with another neurone whose axon crosses (decussates) to the opposite side of the spinal cord.
4. This axon then carries the impulse in the spinothalamic tract to the thalamus in the brain.
5. The spinothalamic tract also conveys temperature sensation as well as pain.
6. The thalamus interacts with higher cortical centres so that the painful stimuli are recognized.

Higher cortical centres can modify the sensation of pain through descending pathways to the thalamus and dorsal horn. Furthermore, pain itself can cause amplification of its own pathway.

As well as the initial stimulation of nociceptors, painful stimuli also often cause the initiation of an inflammatory response, leading to the release of inflammatory mediators from plasma activated by tissue damage and from the nerve terminals themselves. These inflammatory mediators, which include cytokines, prostaglandins, leukotrienes and bradykinin, cause vasodilatation and oedema, as well as stimulate nociceptive pathways themselves, and thus worsen the algesia (pain).

Overall, the inflammatory response can be summarized as follows:

- rubor (redness)
- calor (heat)
- tumor (swelling)
- dolor (pain)
- loss of function.

Analgesia

Different analgesics (pain killers) work by interfering with different parts of the pain pathway. For example, local anaesthetics work by blocking nerve action potentials; non-steroidal anti-inflammatory drugs (NSAIDs) such as aspirin work by inhibiting the production of certain inflammatory mediators (prostaglandins and leukotrienes) via the cyclo-oxygenase (COX) enzyme; opiates such as morphine inhibit the spinal cord dorsal horn (via acting on *mu* receptors) to inhibit the transmission of pain; and alpha$_2$-adrenergic agonists such as tizanidine and clonidine exert their effect by reducing the central transmission of painful stimuli.

Acetaminophen

Acetaminophen (paracetamol) is a peripherally acting drug with no anti-inflammatory activity. It has approximately the same analgesic activity as aspirin and is a useful analgesic and antipyretic (reduces fever). Acetaminophen causes no gastric irritation and is remarkably safe. However, in overdose it can cause liver damage. Up to 4 g daily is the maximum dose for an adult, but acetaminophen toxicity is increased by alcohol, barbiturates and possibly zidovudine.

Non-steroidal anti-inflammatory drugs

NSAIDs are the mainstay of treatment of mild and moderate pain associated with tissue inflammation. Due to their ability to block COX, NSAIDs have analgesic, anti-inflammatory and antipyretic actions.

COX is needed to convert the fatty acid arachidonic acid to prostaglandins, thromboxane and prostacyclin. Prostaglandins cause vasodilatation and increase capillary permeability in areas of inflammation. They also potentiate the algesic effects of inflammatory mediators such as bradykinin, as well as having pyretic effects (via stimulation of interleukin-1). Hence, blocking prostaglandin synthesis with NSAIDs will lead to the three effects described above.

NSAIDs may be irreversible inhibitors of COX (e.g. aspirin) or have reversible effects (e.g. ibuprofen). COX is produced at sites of tissue inflammation and injury in its 'inducible' form, cyclo-oxygenase-2 (COX-2). Thus, it is the inhibition of COX-2 which accounts for the beneficial effects of NSAIDs. However, COX exists in a 'constitutive' form as well, cyclo-oxygenase-1 (COX-1), which produces prostaglandins for housekeeping functions of cells. COX-1 inhibition is responsible for the adverse side effects of some NSAIDs, such as:

- *Gastric ulceration* – prostaglandins have a protective function in inhibiting acid secretion and increasing mucus production in the stomach; thus inhibiting prostaglandin production increases the risk of ulceration.
- *Renal failure* – renal prostaglandins act as vasodilators, and thus without them the renal blood flow is decreased, which can result in worsening renal function and failure
- *Bleeding tendency* – blood platelet function is impaired. One aspirin tablet will reduce platelet function for about 1 week!

Hence, NSAIDs should not be used in patients with renal impairment, those with previous peptic ulcer disease, or those with a bleeding tendency.

Newer COX-2 specific inhibitor drugs (coxibs) which have recently become available (e.g. celecoxib, rofecoxib) offer the promise of the beneficial algesic effects without these unwanted side effects. Indeed, their use has been approved for arthritis and other painful conditions, but their side-effect profile (or lack of it) has yet to be confirmed. 'Hot off the press' studies indicate a possible increase in adverse cardiovascular events with coxibs, leading to the withdrawal of rofecoxib from the market.

A more recent role for NSAIDs in general, and COX-2 inhibitors in particular, is as possible chemoprevention in patients with solid malignancies. Recent epidemiological and histological studies suggest a possible benefit in both primary and secondary prevention in patients with breast, colorectal and prostate cancer, although currently their use in this regard is the subject of much research including that of the first author (P.S.).

Opiates

Opiates exert analgesic actions mainly by blocking *mu* opiate receptors. Opiates bind to their receptors in a stereospecific manner. Most clinically used opiates are of the morphine group (other groups include phenylpiperidine derivatives, methadone derivatives and thebaine derivatives).

Although opiates have profound analgesic effects, they have potentially lethal side effects, and therefore great caution is needed with their use. Acute side effects include:

- respiratory depression
- bradycardia
- altered conscious state (confusion, sedation or euphoria), which is particularly marked in the elderly
- constipation
- pupillary constriction (pinpoint pupils are often a sign of opiate overdose)
- nausea and vomiting (hence an antiemetic should always be given with opiate administration).

Any patient suspected of having opiate-induced respiratory depression that compromises their oxygen saturations (measured with a pulse oximeter) should be given an opiate antagonist such as naloxone to reverse the effect. As the duration of action of naloxone is less than that of most opiates, it should be given as an initial intravenous bolus (typically 400 µg) and then as a continuous infusion.

Opiates have traditionally been given by mouth or intermittent intramuscular injection for postoperative pain relief (e.g. 10 mg up to every 4 hours as needed). This inevitably leads to peaks and troughs in the blood concentrations of the drug, with resultant peaks and troughs in both pain relief and side effects. Continuous repeated small intravenous boluses (e.g. 1 mg up to every 5 min as needed) are becoming more usual therefore, as is the case with patient-controlled analgesia (PCA). PCA also allows patients to control their own analgesia, which in itself leads to decreased analgesic requirement.

Opiates may also be given by anaesthetists via an epidural route (e.g. diamorphine and fentanyl), often in combination with local anaesthetics. This is commonly used for postoperative pain. Transcutaneous opiate administration (e.g. fentanyl patches) has the theoretical advantage of longer duration of action, but its use is limited due to inconsistent absorption of the drug.

Other analgesic agents and methods

There are a multitude of other analgesics on the market, far too numerous to mention. Among them, are clonidine (alpha$_2$-adrenoceptor agonist), ketamine (glutamate agonist) and tramadol (weak opiate agonist). All three drugs have significant side effects and should only be prescribed by anaesthetists.

As well as epidural anaesthesia and PCA, other less traditional methods of pain relief include local anaesthetic blocks (e.g. femoral plexus block for lower limb surgery), cryosurgery to nerves, transcutaneous electrical nerve stimulation (TENS) where non-painful electrical stimuli are applied to the painful region through carbonized rubber electrodes, and cordotomy (sectioning the spinothalamic tracts above the level of the painful lesion). Cryosurgery to the trigeminal nerve can be used to treat neuralgia, at least for a while. TENS is thought to work according to the gate theory of pain, where non-nociceptive stimuli inhibit the central stimulation of painful stimuli arising at the same segmental level. Although TENS can be used in acute pain, it has proved to be much more successful in chronic painful conditions.

Cordotomy may lead to complications from inadvertent damage to nearby descending motor tracts. Also, recurrence of pain, typically after 1 year, is common, and thus cordotomy is usually reserved as a last resort option for patients with pain from malignancy in whom life expectancy is short.

Dental aspects

NSAIDs and acetaminophen (paracetamol) are commonly used to control dental pain and postoperative pain, but it is not recommended that dentists should administer opiates to patients. COX-2 inhibitors are only recommended for patients unable to tolerate conventional NSAIDs. Caution should be exercised if patients have a bleeding tendency, renal impairment or peptic ulcer disease, or are on other medication (Table 1). Depending on the severity of pain, different analgesics are used (see Analgesic ladder; Figure 1).

Table 1 Dental analgesia

Specific analgesics used in dentistry	Interacting drug	Main uses	Possible outcomes
Acetaminophen	Alcohol	Abuse	Liver toxicity
Aspirin	Alcohol	Abuse	Risk of gastrointestinal bleeding
	Hypoglycaemics	Diabetes	Enhanced hypoglycaemia
	Warfarin	Cardiac disease	Risk of gastrointestinal bleeding
NSAIDs	Antihypertensives	Hypertension	Reduced antihypertensive effect
	Lithium	Manic depression	Lithium toxicity
	Methotrexate	Rheumatoid disease	Methotrexate toxicity
	Warfarin	Cardiac disease	Risk of gastrointestinal bleeding

Perioperative pain

- Local analgesia (anaesthesia) should be used wherever possible for outpatient dentistry, with conscious sedation by inhalation (e.g. nitrous oxide and oxygen)

Figure 1 shows the analgesic ladder:

| Severe pain |
| Acetaminophen + strong opioid (morphine) |

| **Moderate pain** |
| Acetaminophen ± weak opioid (codeine, dihydrocodeine or NSAID) |

| **Mild pain** |
| Acetaminophen |

Figure 1 Analgesic ladder

or intravenously (e.g. midazolam), if necessary. Local analgesia (LA) is usually achieved with lidocaine (lignocaine), prilocaine or articaine injected next to the area in question (infiltration anaesthesia) or to block a branch of the trigeminal nerve (regional block anaesthesia).

- General anaesthesia (GA) can be a significant cause of morbidity or even mortality and must be given only in a hospital with critical care facilities.

Five facts

1. The cardinal features of inflammation are heat, redness, pain, swelling and loss of function.
2. The pain pathway can be targeted peripherally or centrally by different classes of analgesics.
3. Opiates can cause respiratory depression and should be used with caution.
4. NSAIDs and acetaminophen (paracetamol) are the mainstay of dental analgesia.
5. Cordotomy is usually a last resort in the management of pain.

Pneumonia

Pneumonia describes a lower respiratory tract infection with radiological changes on chest radiography. It is a potentially dangerous infection with a significant mortality, being a common cause of death in elderly patients. Pneumonia in a previously healthy individual is classed as primary and is usually lobar. Pneumonia secondary to some other disorder is usually bronchopneumonia (patchy areas of infection).

Pneumonia is most common in the elderly, in the immunocompromised and in people at risk of aspiration of material into the lungs, e.g. alcoholics, who can inhale vomit after a binge. Aspiration syndromes involving oral or gastric contents are also associated with gastro-oesophageal reflux disease (GORD), swallowing dysfunction, neurological disorders and structural abnormalities.

Clinical features

The patient with pneumonia may complain of constitutional symptoms of fever, loss of appetite and weight loss. A cough develops, which is usually productive of yellow, green or bloodstained sputum (haemoptysis). Frank coughing up of blood may even occur. The patient may develop shortness of breath. Confusion may occur, especially in the elderly.

There may be clinical signs of lung 'consolidation': i.e. the affected lung may have reduced expansion in inspiration, be dull to percussion, have increased tactile vocal fremitus and have bronchial breathing on auscultation with a stethoscope.

If the pleura become inflamed, pleurisy may develop, when the patient experiences sharp, stabbing localized pain, worse on inspiration and coughing.

Sometimes, a pleural effusion may be present, which may produce stony dull percussion and reduced breath sounds over the effusion.

Pathology

Pneumonia may be classified into community-acquired and hospital-acquired (*nosocomial*) pneumonia and pneumonia in the immunocompromised patient.

Community-acquired pneumonia

Community-acquired pneumonia is the most common form, affecting mainly smokers, the elderly, people with chronic lung disease (e.g. bronchiectasis) and the immuno-suppressed or immunocompromised (see below). These people are also likely to suffer more severe and prolonged illness.

Streptococcus pneumoniae is the most common cause, accounting for about one-third of cases. *Haemophilus influenzae* and pseudomonas tend to cause pneumonia in patients with chronic lung disease. *Staphylococcus aureus* and *Klebsiella* have a tendency to cause cavitating lung lesions and abscesses.

Legionella pneumophila is well known to cause outbreaks of severe pneumonia, arising from sources in a building, e.g. the water tank. Legionnaire's disease was named after an outbreak at an American Legion convention in Philadelphia in 1976. Other causes of bacterial pneumonia include *Chlamydia psittaci* (spread from birds) and *Mycoplasma pneumoniae*.

Viral infections may also cause pneumonia. Influenza, varicella and measles have long been known to cause pneumonia. Human metapneumovirus has recently been identified as a new paramyxovirus in both children and adults. SARS-associated coronavirus (SARS-CoV) has been recognized as causing the recently described severe acute respiratory syndrome (SARS), with a very high mortality.

Hospital-acquired (nosocomial) pneumonia

Any pneumonia developing at least 2 days after hospital admission is deemed a hospital-acquired pneumonia.

Factors which predispose patients to this condition include the following:

- acute illness causing immunosuppression
- invasive procedures such as bronchoscopy, ventilators and intubation, which introduce organisms into the lungs
- sepsis which may lead to haematological spread to the lungs.

The major causes of hospital-acquired pneumonia are Gram-negative bacteria such as pseudomonas, coliforms and MRSA (methicillin-resistant *Staphylococcus aureus*). See chapter on infection control and MRSA.

Pneumonia in the immunocompromised patient

Immunocompromised patients (e.g. AIDS, acute leukaemia, post-chemotherapy) are at risk of infection from the bacterial pathogens described above as well as from less virulent organisms such as viruses (e.g. herpes simplex, cytomegalovirus), fungi (e.g. *Pneumocystis carinii, Candida, Histoplasmosis, Aspergillus*) and tuberculosis.

Complications of pneumonia

Several complications may arise from pneumonia.

Collapse of the affected lobe or segment of lung

This condition is caused by bronchial obstruction with retained mucus, which prevents inflation of the supplied section of lung.

Pneumothorax

Pneumothorax may occur as a result of damage to the lung parenchyma, which leads to leakage of air into the pleural space.

Lung abscess/empyema (abscess in the pleural space)

This condition may occur from extension of the causative organism.

Pleural effusion

Pleural effusion may develop on the side of the affected lung as a result of pleural irritation.

Adult respiratory distress syndrome (ARDS)

ARDS is defined as a refractory hypoxaemia (PaO_2 <8 kPa on at least 50% inspired oxygen) with bilateral pulmonary infiltrates on chest radiograph, in the absence of heart failure. It may be caused by almost any pulmonary injury (as in pneumonia) or systemic injury (e.g. acute pancreatitis).

Investigations

Chest radiograph
A chest radiograph shows consolidation, either in a lobar or diffuse (bronchopneumonia) pattern. There may also be evidence of collapse, pleural effusion or hilar lymphadenopathy.

Arterial blood gas measurement
Arterial blood gases are a measure of hypoxia, and therefore guide oxygen therapy, and carbon dioxide, which is a useful function of ventilation. A rising CO_2 indicates fatigue of the patient's respiratory muscles, and may be an indication for ventilatory support (see below).

Sputum microscopy, culture and sensitivity
Identification of the causative organism is extremely important for the management of pneumonia. Multiple sputum samples should be analysed microscopically using a Gram stain. Culture should also be performed on samples, and the antibiotic sensitivity of any organism isolated in culture assayed. If the patient cannot expectorate, inhaled nebulized saline is sometimes helpful in the production of sputum.

Bronchoscopy with bronchoalveolar lavage
Bronchoscopy with bronchoalveolar lavage has a higher diagnostic yield than sputum examination for the identification of the causative organism and should be performed in pneumonia which is resistant to infection where no organism has been identified.

Blood cultures
Blood cultures should be sent, particularly if the patient is pyrexic.

Serum antigens
Specific assays for antigens to organisms such as *Legionella* and *Mycoplasma* help with the diagnosis.

Serum measurement of cold agglutinins
Cold agglutinins are immunoglobulin M (IgM) autoantibodies to red blood cells, which are most active at 20°C. Their presence is strongly associated with *Mycoplasma* infection.

Management

Oxygen
Oxygen should be given via a mask in order to treat hypoxia. The adequacy of oxygen treatment can be monitored by pulse oximetry and arterial blood gas measurement.

Antibiotics
Antibiotic choice depends on two issues: the clinical setting (e.g. community or hospital) and the identity of the causal organism. Without identification of the organism, initial treatment is empirical and determined by the clinical setting. For community-acquired pneumonia, initial treatment is either with oral *amoxicillin*, or with an oral macrolide such as *erythromycin* or *clarithromycin* if the patient is allergic to penicillins. If the pneumonia is severe (see section below on prognostic markers), then intravenous (IV) co-amoxiclav or cefuroxime plus an IV macrolide should be used.

Once an organism is identified, then antibiotic therapy should be rationalized to optimally treat that pathogen. For example, *Staphylococcus aureus* should be treated with flucloxacillin (if community-acquired) or vancomycin if MRSA is suspected or the pneumonia is hospital-acquired.

Physiotherapy
Physiotherapy is an important aspect of treatment. Exercises and postural manoeuvres aid the drainage of secretions from the affected lung. They also help to prevent alveolar collapse and prevent spread of infection to other parts of the lung.

Ventilatory support
Ventilatory support may be needed if oxygen therapy alone is insufficient to maintain adequate respiratory function. Continuous positive airways pressure (CPAP) is a type of non-invasive ventilation which may be used to prevent alveolar collapse and therefore aid oxygen gas exchange. However, if CPAP is inadequate, or the patient begins to tire, then invasive ventilation in an intensive care setting is most appropriate.

Prophylaxis
Elderly people, together with individuals with chronic respiratory illness or severe non-respiratory illness, should avoid smoking, and should undergo annual vaccination against pneumococcus and influenza.

Prognostic markers in pneumonia
Certain markers have been shown to be predictors of poor prognosis in pneumonia:

- confusion
- urea >7 mmol/L
- respiratory rate greater than 30 breaths per minute
- blood pressure (diastolic) less than 60 mmHg.

Two or more of these markers are associated with a 30 times higher rate of mortality. Such cases should always be treated as 'severe'. Patients should therefore be treated with IV antibiotics (see above) and have a bronchoscopy in order to make the microbiological diagnosis.

Dental aspects

Pneumonia is a severe illness and all but emergency dental treatment should be deferred until recovery.

Further reading

British Thoracic Society. Guidelines for the management of community acquired pneumonia. *Thorax* 2001; 56(suppl IV).

Five facts

1. Pneumonia is a lower respiratory tract infection with changes seen on the chest radiograph.
2. *Streptococcus pneumoniae* is the most common cause of pneumonia.
3. The risk of pneumonia is highest in the elderly, in the immunocompromised and in those predisposed to aspiration (such as alcoholics).
4. Since the organisms which cause community-acquired pneumonia are different to those which cause hospital-acquired (nosocomial) pneumonia, the antibiotics needed to treat them are different.
5. CURB: confusion, urea >7 mmol/L, respiratory rate greater than 30 breaths per minute and diastolic blood pressure less than 60 mmHg are all markers of poor prognosis in pneumonia.

Postoperative complications

No operation is risk-free. Complications can be classified as:

- *local* (specific to the operation site) and *general* (affecting any of the other body systems)
- *immediate* (within the first 24 hours postoperatively), *early* (within the first 4 weeks) and *late* (after 4 weeks postop).

This chapter reviews the general complications of major surgery.

Haemorrhage

It is impossible to make a surgical incision without any bleeding. Appropriate tissue handling, use of diathermy and dressings will help to ensure haemostasis. All patients on warfarin having major surgery should be switched to heparin preoperatively, and some surgical procedures also warrant the cessation of aspirin and clopidogrel therapy (although this practice varies considerably from surgeon to surgeon). The avoidance of significant haemorrhage not only decreases the risk of postoperative shock but it also reduces wound infection rates and leads to quicker patient convalescence. The 'cut and run' surgical approach of cavalier surgeons should be replaced with careful, meticulous attention to haemostasis.

Wound infection

Any operation can become infected, since epithelia are broken and/or foreign instrumentation is introduced. In cases with preoperative sepsis, postoperative infection rates are high.

Meticulous attention to sterility and tissue handling are imperative to prevent infections as much as possible. All sites of potential infection should be carefully debrided and dressed appropriately. The commonest organisms for postoperative infection are penicillin-resistant *Staphylococcus aureus*, *Streptococcus faecalis*, pseudomonads, coliforms and *Bacteroides (Porphyromonas)*.

Infections can be due to preoperative, operative or postoperative factors. Preoperative factors include pre-existing infection or contamination, e.g. perforated appendix, open fracture. Operative factors include non-sterilization of instruments and surgeons' hands, and poor surgical tissue handling. Meticulous attention to sterility and tissue handling are imperative to prevent infections as much as possible. All sites of potential infection should be carefully debrided and dressed appropriately. Postoperative factors are usually cross-infection from infected patients on the same ward or nurses during dressing changes. Even clinical white coats have been shown to increase postoperative wound infection rates.

Typically, wound infections (surgical site infections) occur around day 5 after the operation, but may present later if antibiotics have been used. The characteristic signs of inflammation are present at the wound site:

- dolor (pain)
- calor (heat)

- rubor (redness)
- tumor (swelling).

The patient may also exhibit systemic features of infection:

- malaise
- anorexia
- vomiting
- swinging pyrexia.

Release of sutures or surgical clips may allow pus to escape and aid resolution of the infection.

Management
The importance of scrupulous theatre and dressing technique cannot be stressed enough. Also, isolation of infected cases and eliminating carriers with colds or septic lesions among the medical and nursing staff is important. Hand washing is the single most important thing that ward staff can do to minimize the risk of infection in their surgical patients.

Established infection is treated by antibiotics if it is cellulitis, and drainage if there is pus. Antibiotics do not treat pus.

Antibiotic prophylaxis
In some cases it is appropriate to give antibiotics prophylactically before a surgical procedure. The choice of regime is tailored according to the most likely bacteria that need targeting, and individual protocols vary between hospitals and are dependent on the local circumstances. Whatever antibiotic regime is used, it will be useless unless adequate drug levels are reached in the circulation at the time of exposure to infection (i.e. during surgery).

Common examples requiring prophylaxis are now considered.

Valvular heart disease
Patients with valvular heart disease are given prophylaxis against haematogenous bacterial colonization of the valve that results in infective endocarditis. This is especially true for patients with rheumatic mitral valve disease, as blood flows quicker through the mitral valve than any other heart valve, predisposing it to colonization.

Presence of a foreign body
In prosthetic joint replacements (hip replacements are one of the commonest operations performed in the NHS), antibiotic prophylaxis is given to prevent prosthetic infection at the time of implantation. The usual culprit is *Staphylococcus aureus*, and thus antibiotic cover must include combating this organism. Infection of the prosthesis can lead to prosthetic failure, joint destruction, osteomyelitis and septicaemia, and can therefore be extremely serious.

Transplant surgery
Transplant patients are immunosuppressed and thus need antibiotic prophylaxis to prevent infection.

Contaminated wounds
Wounds are classified as clean (<2% risk of infection), clean-contaminated (2–10% risk of infection), contaminated (10–30% risk of infection) and dirty (>30% risk of infection). Contaminated and dirty wounds (e.g. gangrene of ischaemic limb, dog bite wound, perforated bowel, open fractures, operations that open body cavities especially the large bowel) require antibiotic prophylaxis. In colonic surgery, antibiotics that cover anaerobes (e.g. metronidazole) are needed.

MRSA (see also chapter on infection control and MRSA)
Staphylococcus aureus is commonly carried on the skin or in the nose of healthy people. Approximately 25–30% of the population is colonized in the nose at a given time. Many *Staphylococcus aureus* strains have become resistant to various antibiotics, including penicillinase-resistant antibiotics (flucloxacillin), and are therefore called methicillin- or preferably multi-resistant *Staphylococcus aureus*, or MRSA (methicillin has long been discontinued).

MRSA can cause exactly the same kinds of infection as staphylococci in general and can spread by close contact with infected people, almost always by direct physical contact, and not through the air. Spread may also be by indirect contact by touching objects (towels, sheets, wound dressings, clothes, workout areas, sports equipment) contaminated by the infected skin of a person with MRSA.

Risk factors for MRSA include prolonged hospital stay, receiving broad-spectrum antibiotics, being hospitalized in an intensive care or burn unit, spending time close to other patients with MRSA, having recent surgery or carrying MRSA in the nose without developing illness. MRSA infections are thus more common among hospitalized patients who are elderly, sick or who have an open wound (such as a bedsore) or a urinary or intravenous (IV) catheter.

MRSA infections can be prevented by the following guidelines:

- avoid contact with wounds or material contaminated from wounds
- follow good hygiene procedures
- if hands are not visibly soiled, use an alcohol-based waterless antiseptic agent for routinely decontaminating hands
- when hands are visibly dirty or contaminated with proteineous material such as blood, wash hands thoroughly with a non-antimicrobial soap and water, or an antimicrobial soap and water
- keep cuts and abrasions clean and covered with a proper dressing until healed
- use a moisturizer to prevent skin cracking.

Vancomycin-resistant bacteria
Vancomycin-resistant *Staphylococcus aureus* (VRSA) infections and vancomycin-resistant enterococcus (VRE) are starting to appear.

Antibiotic-associated enterocolitis
Broad-spectrum antibiotics such as cephalosporins (e.g. cefotaxime) and clindamycin destroy the normal commensal gut flora and select out resistant strains, such as the toxin-producing *Clostridium difficile* (previously known as *Cl. welchii*). The toxins produce mucosal inflammation and pseudomembrane formation (so-called

pseudomembranous colitis), causing watery diarrhoea. This typically presents within the first week after antibiotic use, with loss of fluid and resultant shock, and sometimes a toxic dilatation of the colon.

Management is supportive with IV fluid and electrolyte replacement, withdrawing the offending antibiotic, starting metronidazole or vancomycin, and keeping the patient nil by mouth until improvement.

Pulmonary collapse and chest infection

Almost all abdominal and thoracic operations will result in some degree of lung collapse within the first few postoperative hours. This is as a result of increased mucus retention that occurs from surgery. The mucus retention causes blocking of distal bronchioles, resulting in the collapse of the supplied lung segments. The collapsed lung segment (usually basal, due to the effects of gravity and the ventilation/perfusion gradients in different regions of the lungs) may become secondarily infected by inhaled or aspirated organisms, leading to chest infection (typically around 1 week postop). Rarely, lung abscess may result. Typical signs of chest infection include dyspnoea, tachycardia, pyrexia, cyanosis and difficulty coughing. Physiotherapy may aid the expectoration of sputum. Purulent sputum is a clear sign of chest infection, and warrants culture and antibiotic treatment.

Risk factors for this complication are:

- Preoperative:
  - pre-existing lung infection
  - smoking
  - chronic lung disease (e.g. chronic obstructive pulmonary disease)
  - ankylosing spondylosis and other conditions impairing chest wall movement and therefore ventilation.
- Operative:
  - general anaesthetic (GA) drugs (decrease cilia movement and thus increase mucus retention)
  - type of surgery (e.g. diaphragmatic hernia repair, thoracic surgery, abdominal surgery).
- Postoperative:
  - pain (impairs ventilation).

Patients deemed to be at high risk of chest infection may be considered for pre- and post-operative breathing exercises and prophylactic antibiotics. Elective surgery should not be performed in patients with active chest infection. In certain cases of major surgery in high-risk individuals, a period of preoperative optimization with supranormal oxygenation is given in the intensive care unit.

The single most important preventative measure that patients can do to decrease their risk of postoperative chest infection is to stop smoking at least 2 weeks before the operation.

Thromboembolic disease

This subject is dealt with separately in the chapter on thromboembolic disease.

Postoperative pyrexia

There are many causes of a fever after surgery. Surgery itself stimulates an acute inflammatory response, with the release of pyrogenic cytokines such as interleukin-1. Hence, a pyrexia within the first 24 hours postop is often normal. Continued pyrexia, especially of swinging nature, is an indication of infection.

The differential diagnosis includes:

- wound infection
- cannula site infection
- chest infection
- thromboembolic disease
- urinary tract infection (UTI)
- enterocolitis
- gastroenteritis
- drug reaction
- deep-seated abscess (e.g. pelvic abscess after abdominal or pelvic surgery).

Dental aspects

The development of a surgical site infection (SSI) is suggested by features such as:

- pus draining from the wound
- the wound becoming excessively tender
- pain or swelling increasing 48 hours after the wound was made
- increasing redness around the wound (cellulitis)
- a red streak from the wound toward the heart (lymphangitis)
- the lymph node draining that area becoming large and tender (lymphadenitis)
- fever
- wound failing to heal within 10 days after the injury
- the scab increasing in size
- a pimple or yellow crust forming on the wound (impetigo).

Most odontogenic infections are polymicrobial but anaerobes generally outnumber aerobes by at least four-fold. Anaerobic bacteria are important as part of the normal oral flora and include Gram-positive cocci and bacilli as well as Gram-negative bacilli. Representative species include *Porphyromonas* (*Bacteroides*), *Fusobacterium*, *Peptostreptococcus*, *Actinomyces* and *Prevotella*.

Most odontogenic and orofacial infections respond to drainage, either by endodontic treatment, incision or tooth extraction. Analgesics may also be required.

Most odontogenic and orofacial infections respond well to penicillin or metronidazole, but increasing rates of resistance due to production of beta-lactamases have lowered the usefulness of penicillins. Co-amoxiclav and clindamycin, because of their broad spectrum of activity and resistance to beta-lactamase, are increasingly often used as first-line drugs.

Fascial space infections of the neck are dangerous since they can embarrass the airway, erode the carotid vessels, cause toxicity, or spread to the mediastinum or intracranially. Fascial space infections usually arise from the oral flora, are polymicrobial and involve predominantly anaerobes, including Gram-positive cocci and bacilli as well as Gram-negative bacilli. Patients with fascial space infections must be admitted for hospital care, which may involve drainage and usually high-dose antibiotics.

Infections of prosthetic joints are usually due to non-oral organisms such as staphylococci and only exceptionally rarely to oral bacteria. Even where viridans streptococci have been found in infected joints, they could have come from non-oral sources, or simply have come from a bacteraemia associated with chewing.

Antibiotic prophylaxis is therefore not indicated for dental surgery on most patients with bone pins, plates and screws or with total joint replacements. However, antibiotic prophylaxis before dental treatment that is likely to initiate a bacteraemia may be considered where dental at-risk procedures are to be carried out:

- in patients who have recent new joints (within 2 years)
- in haemophiliacs
- where the joint has previously been infected
- where the patient is immunocompromised, such as patients with diabetes or rheumatoid disease.

Five facts

1. Postoperative complications can be classified into local (specific) and general.
2. Complications can also be divided into immediate (within 24 hours), early (within 4 weeks) or late (after 4 weeks).
3. Infection and bleeding are potential complications of virtually any surgical intervention.
4. Chest infection, UTI and thromboembolic disease are common causes of a postoperative pyrexia.
5. Antibiotic prophylaxis is indicated for dental surgery in patients at high risk of developing infection (e.g. recent new joints, haemophiliacs, immunocompromised, diabetics).

Principles of management of cancer

Cancer treatment can be with surgery, radiotherapy, chemotherapy (cytotoxic drugs singly or in combination), stem cell transplantation, immunotherapy (monoclonal antibodies and – on the horizon – vaccines), and now gene therapy. Hormonal treatments and palliative care are also very important.

Surgery

Surgery is usually for curative intent in the management of operable malignancy. The principles are that the tumour should be removed with a margin of normal tissue, and that dissemination of the tumour should be avoided as much as possible. Often, lymph nodes are removed, either as part of the curative operation, or for staging purposes. Traditionally surgical approaches for cancer were open but, increasingly, laparoscopic approaches are being used in certain malignancies, e.g. colon, prostate.

Occasionally, surgical approaches are palliative. This may be to reduce tumour bulk and thus decrease local effects of the tumour, e.g. neurosurgery for brain tumours causing mass effects. Also in certain cases of incurable gastrointestinal malignancies, palliative surgery can 'bypass' the tumour to allow continued oral intake.

Chemotherapy

Chemotherapy is used mainly to damage or destroy proliferating malignant cells, particularly in malignant disease affecting blood cells, and lymphomas, but also for some more solid tumours. The main problem is that these agents cannot differentiate between malignant and normal cells, and thus damage normally proliferating cells, such as bone marrow, gastrointestinal epithelium and hair follicles. This is what causes their potentially severe side effects:

- bone marrow depression (and consequent immunosuppression and infection)
- nausea and vomiting
- alopecia (hair loss)
- mucositis

There are four main classes of chemotherapeutic agent:

1. *Alkylating agents*, which work by either preventing cell division by covalently cross-linking the two strands of DNA, or by reacting with DNA base pairs. Examples include cyclophosphamide and cisplatin.
2. *Anti-metabolites*, which interfere with DNA synthesis. Examples include methotrexate and 5-fluorouracil.
3. *Antibiotics*, which intercalate between base pairs and prevent RNA production. Examples include doxorubicin and mitomycin.
4. *Vinca alkaloids*, which inhibit mitosis by preventing spindle formation. Examples include vincristine and vinblastine.

Radiotherapy

Ionizing radiation used in clinical practice for the killing of cancerous cells may be either particulate (e.g. electrons, protons, neutrons, *alpha* particles) or electromagnetic (e.g. X-rays, *gamma* rays). Radiotherapy causes high-energy interactions between molecules. This causes DNA damage via release of kinetic energy. This may trigger apoptosis (programmed cell death) or cause chromosomal abnormalities that prevent mitosis. Hence, cells may not appear abnormal until they attempt to divide. As malignant cells usually spend a greater proportion of their cell cycles in mitosis, radiotherapy will kill them preferentially. However, slow-growing tumours may not respond or respond only slowly to radiotherapy.

Even so, normal cell killing does still occur to some extent, which leads to side effects dependent on the tissue irradiated. For example, oesophageal irradiation can cause oesophagitis and stricture formation, whereas lymphoedema is common after axillary node irradiation for breast cancer. The treatment can also damage the developing fetus if used in pregnancy.

The ability of radiotherapy to cure a tumour depends on its size, radiosensitivity and the tolerance of the surrounding normal tissue (as this affects the doses that can be given). Radiotherapy can be given as primary treatment or pre- (adjuvant) or post-operatively (i.e. adjuvant treatment), either to aid cure or as palliation. Common preoperative indications include downstaging tumours and reducing risk of intra-operative seeding of malignant cells (e.g. rectal cancer). Common palliative reasons are to relieve symptoms (e.g. pain, risk of fracture) from bony metastases.

Radiotherapy can be given systemically (e.g. iodine-131 for thyroid cancer), it can be implanted into the tissue being treated (e.g. brachytherapy for tongue and prostate cancer), or it can be given as external beam fractionated sources, with several doses given over several weeks.

Hormonal treatments

Certain cancers are dependent on an endocrine axis for their progress, and thus can be treated by hormonal manipulations. Common examples include the use of anti-androgens and LHRH (luteinizing hormone-releasing hormone) analogues for prostate cancer, tamoxifen for breast cancer and thyroxine for thyroid cancer.

Palliative care

Patients with cancer should be made as comfortable as possible during the terminal phase of their disease. Specific issues that may arise include pain management, nutrition and feeding, management of treatment side effects, psychological support and family concerns. A multi-disciplinary approach involving a range of specialists is preferred, but the palliative care physician should assume overall control.

Dental aspects

A variety of approaches are used in the management of oral cancer:

- surgery

- radiotherapy
- chemotherapy (occasionally).

Radiotherapy and cytotoxic chemotherapy can have profound adverse effects on oral health and quality of life and can give rise to the major complaints of the patient undergoing cancer treatment, especially when the radiotherapy field affects the head and neck and involves the oral cavity and salivary glands (Table 1).

Table 1 Complications of oral radiotherapy

Complications

Nausea	Taste changes	Tooth hypersensitivity
Vomiting	Infections	Trismus
Mucositis	Caries	Osteoradionecrosis
Dry mouth	Pulp pain and necrosis	Craniofacial defects

Five facts

1. Surgery is the commonest curative modality for most cancers.
2. Radiotherapy and chemotherapy may be used in an adjuvant, neoadjuvant, curative or palliative setting.
3. Chemotherapy inhibits cell proliferation and therefore often has severe side effects (e.g. nausea, vomiting, alopecia, bone marrow depression).
4. Radiotherapy kills dividing cells and therefore is often less effective against slow-growing tumours.
5. Radiotherapy to the oral cavity can cause mucositis, dry mouth and osteo-radionecrosis.

Principles of neoplasia

Definitions

Not all disorders of growth are malignant (cancer). Before we deal with cancer, we should first understand the various disorders of growth:

- *Hyperplasia* – increase in number of cells, usually as a result of inflammation, increased workload, excess endocrine drive or increased metabolic demand. Examples include renal hyperplasia and benign prostatic hyperplasia.
- *Hypertrophy* – increase in size of cells, usually as a response to a need for increased function. Examples include increased skeletal volume in athletes, and pregnant uterus. It may occur in conjunction with hyperplasia, e.g. benign prostatic hypertrophy/hyperplasia.
- *Metaplasia* – the reversible replacement of one cell type for another, usually as an adaptive response to chronic irritation. Examples include squamous metaplasia in the airways (change from columnar epithelium) and adenomatous metaplasia in Barrett's oesophagus (change from squamous epithelium). Metaplasia is often associated with an increased risk of malignant transformation via dysplasia (see below).
- *Dysplasia* – disordered cell development with increased mitosis and pleomorphism. This is usually preneoplastic, with many cancers such as oral cancer being preceded by it.
- *Neoplasia* – abnormal mass of tissue with uncoordinated and increased growth persisting beyond any causative stimuli. In other words, the important point about cancer is that it has escaped the body's regulating mechanisms such as apoptosis (programmed cell death).

Cancer

Malignant neoplasms are a leading cause of morbidity and mortality in middle-aged people or the elderly. Solid tumours are most common in the lung, breast, colon, cervix, stomach, pancreas, ovary and prostate in adults and most are carcinomas. Tobacco is at least partly responsible for many of these malignant neoplasms. Younger people may be affected by haematological malignancies and occasionally rare tumours. The prognosis of much malignant disease is poor and treatment can have significant adverse effects; thus, prevention and early detection of lesions is important.

Cancer stage and grade
Stage
The stage of a cancer refers to its size and spread. The most common staging system used universally for most tumours is the TNM classification:

T = tumour size
N = lymph node involvement
M = presence of metastases

Other commonly used classifications are the Manchester system for breast carcinoma (see chapter on breast cancer) and the Dukes' system for colorectal carcinoma (see chapter on colorectal cancer).

Grade

The grade of a cancer refers to its degree of differentiation, i.e. how similar it is to its tissue of origin. The degree of differentiation usually corresponds to how aggressive the tumour is, with less differentiated tumours classically being more aggressive. Features of poor differentiation include:

- increased nuclear pleomorphism
- atypical mitoses
- hyperchromatic nuclei
- increased nuclear:cytoplasmic ratio
- giant cells.

There are many different grading systems but the commonest is:

G1 = well differentiated
G2 = moderately differentiated
G3 = poorly/un-differentiated

What stimulates cancer formation (carcinogenesis)?

Cancer arises from genetic mutation or damage to a single cell (monoclonal cell theory), or from an inherited germ line defect with subsequent damage after its carriage into a daughter cell (Knudson's two-hit hypothesis).

There are four types of genes that can be affected to produce a cancer:

1. proto-oncogenes (if mutated these genes are up-regulated to oncogenes that promote growth)
2. tumour suppressor genes or anti-oncogenes (these genes suppress growth, and thus, if mutated, their action is diminished)
3. pro-apoptotic genes (these genes cause programmed cell death, and thus, when mutated, the cancer escapes apoptosis)
4. DNA repair genes (these genes excise mutated gene segments and are down-regulated in neoplasia).

The effect of mutation of any or all of these genes is clonal expansion of the tissue mass, which after an additional mutation (second-hit) leads to malignant transformation.

The mutagens that can start off this process can be divided into:

- chemical (e.g. hundreds of substances in tobacco and cigarette smoke, asbestos, polycyclic aromatic hydrocarbons)
- physical (e.g. ultraviolet light, ionizing radiation)
- viruses (e.g. hepatitis B virus, Epstein–Barr virus, human papillomaviruses).

How does the cancer progress?

The speed of tumour cell growth varies from tumour to tumour and depends on the proportion of cells in the replication phases of the cell cycle. However, as all tumours get larger they need nutrients to survive, and thus they need to form their own network of blood vessels (known as tumour neovascularization or angiogenesis). Most tumours start this process once >1–2 mm diameter. Angiogenic factors are secreted by the tumour cells (e.g. vascular endothelial growth factor – VEGF) and anti-angiogenic factors are inhibited (e.g. angiostatin). The process of angiogenesis is not fully understood and a variety of other cell signalling pathways also regulate it.

Cancers also invade locally and spread distantly (metastasize); in fact, this is what distinguishes benign from malignant tumours. For local invasion, cells must break free of each other (loss of cell-to-cell adhesion, often due to down-regulation of E-cadherin), and invade through the basement membrane (often via increased laminin receptor binding and protease secretion). Once tumour cells have reached the circulation, they then disseminate to distant sites and coalesce together at such sites after extravasating through the transporting vessels. At the metastatic sites the tumour mass must once again stimulate angiogenesis for survival. Different tumours have different preferential sites for metastasis; e.g. lung cancer typically metastasizes to kidney and liver, whereas prostate cancer typically goes to bone.

Tumour markers
These substances found in blood are secreted in certain malignancies, and thus can be used clinically to monitor the progress of those cancers. Examples include prostate-specific antigen (PSA) for prostate cancer, carcinoembryonic antigen (CEA) for colorectal carcinoma and *alpha*-fetoprotein (AFP) for hepatocellular carcinoma.

Prostate-specific antigen
PSA has revolutionized the diagnosis and management of prostate cancer, but it is also elevated in non-malignant prostatic disorders such as prostatitis, benign prostatic hyperplasia and prostatic infarction. PSA may also be elevated after prostatic trauma, resulting from a prostatic biopsy or an overzealous digital rectal examination.

Carcinoembryonic antigen
CEA is elevated in over two-thirds of cases of colorectal cancer, but it also rises in cirrhosis, alcoholic hepatitis and inflammatory bowel disease. Unlike PSA, it is not sensitive or specific enough to be used in screening, and thus the use of CEA is limited to monitor the efficacy of therapy and the detection of colorectal cancer recurrence.

Alpha-fetoprotein
AFP is also elevated in cirrhosis, chronic hepatitis, pregnancy and non-seminomatous germ cell tumours of the testes. Its use, therefore, is again limited to monitoring treatment effects and the diagnosis of recurrence.

Dental aspects

Oral cancer is usually squamous cell carcinoma (OSCC). Common sites are the lips, the lateral border of the tongue and the floor of the mouth. OSCC is mainly a disease of the elderly, and high rates are seen particularly in India, Sri Lanka and Brazil.

Predisposing factors include:

- Sun-exposure: lower lip cancer, especially in white races, in sunny climates, in persons frequently exposed to the sun and after transplant immunosuppression.
- Tobacco: smoked and/or chewed.
- Alcohol.
- Betel (*Areca*) use, as in betel chewing.
- Immunosuppression.

A diet rich in fresh fruit and vegetables appears to have some protective effect.

Five facts

1. Cancer is a condition of uncontrolled growth and proliferation that persists beyond any causative stimuli.
2. Cancer arises from a genetic mutation or damage to a single cell, or from an inherited germ line defect with subsequent damage after its carriage into a daughter cell.
3. The incidence of most cancers increases with age.
4. Smoking is a major risk factor for many cancers.
5. Oral cancer is usually of squamous origin and is common in the Indian subcontinent due to betel chewing.

Prostate cancer

Prostate cancer is increasing in incidence as the general health of the population improves and people are tending to live longer. Prostate cancer is the most common tumour in men over 60 years old, and 80% of men aged 80 years old have it, although they may not be aware of it nor may it be of any clinical significance. This is because prostate cancer is the slowest growing solid malignancy, and so many patients die *with it* rather than *from it*.

Risk factors for prostate cancer include a family history of prostate cancer and race; it is considerably more common in those of African descent. Diets high in animal fat may possibly raise the risk and diets high in fruits and vegetables may lower the risk. Benign prostatic hypertrophy (BPH) does *not* seem to increase the chances of getting prostate cancer.

Pathology

Prostate cancer is usually adenocarcinoma. Spread can occur locally to periprostatic tissues and adjacent organs (e.g. seminal vesicles, bladder, urethra, rectum), via lymphatics to iliac and para-aortic nodes, and via the bloodstream to bone (typically, sites of red marrow such as the pelvis, spine, ribs and skull). The characteristic feature of the bone metastases is that they are usually osteosclerotic (appear more dense on X-ray) rather than osteolytic (appear as a defect on X-ray).

Lung and liver metastases can also occur but are less common than with breast, kidney, lung or colorectal tumours (the other common solid malignancies).

Clinical features

Cancer tends to occur in the periphery of the prostate, and thus obstructs urination less commonly than does benign disease, which typically affects the transitional and central zones. Thus features such as poor stream, hesitancy, incomplete emptying, frequency and nocturia are uncommon and many patients with prostate cancer present asymptomatically after screening tests (discussed below) are found to be abnormal.

Investigations

Serum prostate-specific antigen (PSA) assay followed by digital rectal examination (DRE) are standard investigations. It is important to note that DRE alone is very unreliable in detecting or excluding prostate cancer, and that all patients being examined for prostate cancer should have their PSA levels checked **before** DRE.

Like all cancers, prostate tumours are staged using the TNM system, but the important point is that the cancer can be confined to the prostate (so-called early prostate cancer) or may have invaded outside the gland (so-called advanced prostate cancer).

Suspected cases of prostate cancer should have a transrectal ultrasound scan of the prostate (TRUS) plus biopsy to confirm the diagnosis if treatment is to be contemplated. Once the diagnosis is confirmed histologically, it is important to attempt to stage the cancer. Unfortunately, bone scans and magnetic resonance imaging (MRI) scans are poor at doing this. A PSA <10 µg/L, a low-grade tumour on TRUS biopsy (a so-called Gleason score <7) and a tumour where the nodule feels confined to the gland on DRE are good predictors that the cancer is organ-confined (early prostate cancer).

Treatment

As the risk of dying from early prostate cancer after 10–15 years is roughly 25%, only patients with a life expectancy of >10 years are usually offered curative treatment, although this is controversial. It becomes very difficult to know which patients need treatment and which will die of something else before their prostate cancer becomes significant.

Early prostate cancer is potentially curable, whereas advanced disease is not. In patients with early prostate cancer, curative treatment may be attempted (e.g. radical prostatectomy, external beam radiotherapy or brachytherapy – a form of surgically delivered radiotherapy). All such treatments have a cure rate of roughly 85% at 10–15 years but, as stated earlier, only one-quarter of these patients will die of their prostate cancer in this time period.

In patients with advanced prostate cancer, the aim is to control the disease as much as possible, and since prostate cancer is testosterone-dependent, hormonal treatments are used (such as anti-androgens, luteinizing hormone-releasing hormone (LHRH) agonists or even orchiectomy).

Prognosis

As stated earlier, patients with early prostate cancer have an extremely good prognosis, even without treatment in many cases. Unfortunately, the 12% of patients who present with metastatic disease have an extremely poor prognosis, with most patients becoming hormone resistant after a variable time.

The problem is that there is no way currently of knowing which patients with early disease are likely to develop significant disease, which of them are likely to relapse after curative treatment and which of those patients with metastatic disease are likely to develop hormone resistance, and when all these events may occur.

Prevention and screening

PSA testing has meant that many more cases of prostate cancer are being diagnosed at an early stage. PSA followed by DRE is recommended annually for men over 50 years old in the USA. Screening for prostate cancer has not yet been formally recommended in the UK, although men who ask to have their PSA measured cannot be refused.

Dental aspects

Metastases occasionally involve the jaw and are typically osteosclerotic.

Five facts

1. Prostate cancer is the commonest tumour in men >60 years old in the UK.
2. PSA has revolutionized the detection of prostate cancer.
3. Many men die *with* prostate cancer rather than *from* prostate cancer.
4. Curative options for prostate cancer include surgery, conformal external beam radiotherapy and brachytherapy.
5. Osteosclerotic metastases can occur in the jaw.

Renal disease

This chapter is divided into sections on renal failure, urinary tract calculi (stones), renal neoplasms (tumours) and dental aspects of renal disease.

Renal failure

Loss of renal function results in a reduced glomerular filtration rate or GFR (renal failure) and may be caused by:

- *pre-renal conditions* such as renal hypoperfusion in severe shock or haemorrhage
- *intrinsic renal disease* such as trauma, disease or drug damage
- *post-renal disorders* such as obstruction of renal outflow by calculi, prostatic hypertrophy or tumour.

Renal failure can come on suddenly (acute renal failure or ARF). However, renal failure more usually develops slowly (chronic renal failure or CRF).

Acute renal failure

ARF describes an acute impairment of renal function, defined arbitrarily, by a *serum creatinine >200 µmol/L*. Biochemical abnormalities include:

- raised creatinine and urea
- hyperkalaemia, which may be life-threatening due to risk of cardiac arrest
- acidosis, which may cause confusion and drowsiness.

Patients may also present with nausea, vomiting and tiredness. Most cases of ARF are associated with decreased urine output (oliguria) or no urine output (anuria). In these patients symptoms of volume overload are present, e.g. ankle oedema and shortness of breath (caused by pulmonary oedema). *By far the most common causes of ARF are pre-renal conditions.*

Chronic renal failure

CRF refers to long-term, irreversible renal impairment, which (like ARF) is arbitrarily defined as a serum creatinine >200 µmol/L. It may sometimes arise from failure to recover renal function following ARF. Alternatively, CRF may arise insidiously. In the UK, the main causes of CRF include:

- diabetes mellitus (30%)
- hypertension (20%)
- renal artery stenosis
- glomerulonephritis
- tubulo-interstitial nephritis
- vasculitis, e.g. SLE (systemic lupus erythematosus).

Complications of CRF
Anaemia
Renal disease leads to reduced erythropoietin secretion (the hormone which would normally stimulate the bone marrow to produce red blood cells), and CRF itself leads

to an anaemia of chronic disease. Normocytic normochromic anaemia is thus produced, which may be treated with regular injections of erythropoietin. Blood transfusions may also be needed.

Vascular disease
Atherosclerosis, with consequent ischaemic heart disease, cerebrovascular disease and peripheral vascular disease, occurs mainly as a consequence of hypertension. Aggressive treatment of all cardiovascular risk factors is therefore extremely important.

Renal osteodystrophy
Inadequate hydroxylase activity by the kidney to convert the vitamin D metabolite 25-hydroxycholecalciferol to 1,25-dihydroxycholecalciferol leads to low plasma calcium levels. The low calcium of osteomalacia leads to *secondary hyperparathyroidism*. In secondary hyperparathyroidism, the parathyroid hormone (PTH) acts to mobilize bone stores and decrease renal excretion of calcium, in order to raise low serum calcium levels. The combination of osteomalacia and secondary hyperparathyroidism therefore combines to cause further bone disease. Sometimes, the response of the parathyroid glands may be excessive, which leads to *tertiary hyperparathyroidism*. Vitamin D and calcium supplements are therefore given to treat (and prevent) hyperparathyroidism and osteomalacia.

Pericarditis and pericardial effusion
Pericarditis and pericardial effusion are also complications of CRF.

Bleeding
Uraemia (raised serum urea) inhibits platelet function and therefore prolongs the bleeding time. However, the coagulation pathway is not affected, which explains why the activated partial thromboplastin time (APTT) and prothrombin time (PT) are unchanged (see chapter on bleeding tendency).

Causes of intrinsic renal disease
Damage to the glomerulus (glomerulonephritis), the tubule or interstitium (tubulo-interstitial nephritis), renal arteries (reno-vascular disease) or an abnormality in the structure of the kidneys may all cause intrinsic renal disease. Although these causes of renal disease are discussed below, please remember that most causes of renal failure are due to pre-renal and post-renal failure (see ARF).

Glomerulonephritis (GN)
Minimal change GN
Minimal change GN typically presents as the *nephrotic syndrome* (oedema and proteinuria). Minimal change disease accounts for most cases of nephrotic syndrome in children, but may occur at any age. Nephrotic syndrome is associated with a loss of *>3 g protein* in the urine over 24 hours. The consequent hypoalbuminaemia causes oedema, and changes in clotting factors and dehydration produces a high risk of thrombosis. Factor VIII, fibrinogen and other clotting factors are raised, with loss of antithrombin III, leading to a hypercoagulable state. Light microscopy of the

glomerulus appears normal but electron microscopy reveals fusion of the podocytes (foot processes of the glomerular cells).

Membranous GN
Membranous GN is the most common cause of nephrotic syndrome in adults. Histology reveals a thickened glomerular basement membrane (GBM). It may be primary (idiopathic), but is also associated with drugs (such as methotrexate, penicillamine and gold) and heavy metals.

Rapidly progressive/crescentic GN (RPGN)
RPGN usually presents with the *nephritic syndrome*. In the nephritic syndrome, patients have oliguria, haematuria and proteinuria and may have features of volume overload, such as hypertension, pulmonary oedema, peripheral oedema and a raised jugular venous pressure (JVP). The main cause of RPGN is an immune response to streptococcal infection (usually pharyngitis). Histology may show necrotic tissue, leading to the formation of crescents in the glomerulus.

Mesangiocapillary GN (MCGN)
MCGN usually presents with proteinuria and sometimes haematuria. MCGN is most commonly associated with hepatitis B and C infections.

Immunoglobulin A (IgA) nephritis
IgA nephritis normally presents with haematuria, with or without proteinuria. Episodes may follow acute respiratory tract infection, as with RPGN. There is a strong association with Henoch–Schönlein purpura, which is a systemic vasculitis causing a purpuric rash and abdominal pain. Glomerular IgA deposition may be seen using immunofluorescence.

Focal segmental glomerulosclerosis
Focal segmental glomerulosclerosis presents with the nephritic syndrome of proteinuria. It may be primary, or associated with other conditions such as heroin misuse or HIV infection.

Systemic vasculitis
Numerous systemic vasculitides such as polyarteritis nodosa (PAN), Wegener's granulomatosis and SLE may all cause glomerulonephritis. PAN is associated with the presence of perinuclear antineutrophil cytoplasmic antibody (pANCA). Wegener's granulomatosis is associated with the presence of cytoplasmic ANCA (cANCA).

Anti-glomerular basement membrane disease is a very rare disorder which causes rapidly progressive GN and pulmonary haemorrhage. It does this by direct immune damage by IgG to Type IV collagen in the glomerular basement membrane (GBM) and lung parenchyma.

Tubulo-interstitial nephritis
Tubulo-interstitial nephritis describes inflammation in the tubule and/or interstitium (extracellular space) surrounding the tubule. In practice, agents which cause glomerulonephritis also cause a certain degree of tubulo-interstitial nephritis, but some conditions in particular are associated with it.

Drugs
Drugs are the most common cause of tubulo-interstitial nephritis. Non-steroidal anti-inflammatory drugs (NSAIDs) and penicillins are among the many drugs which are associated with it.

Infections
Acute or chronic pyelonephritis leads to interstitial inflammation. Other infections such as tuberculosis (TB) and leptospirosis are also associated with the disease.

Toxins
Toxins such as lead, some herbal medications and certain mushrooms are associated with the disease.

Immune/inflammatory
Multiple myeloma (see haematological malignancies) produces light chains that may cause a tubular nephritis. Inflammatory diseases such as sarcoidosis and SLE may also cause tubulo-interstitial disease.

Reno-vascular disease
Renal artery stenosis
Renal artery stenosis is the most common cause of reno-vascular disease (see chapter on hypertension).

Thrombotic microangiopathy
Thrombotic microangiopathy is a condition characterized by damage to small blood vessels, with subsequent thrombus formation and platelet/fibrin consumption. The passage of blood through these damaged vessels leads to the physical destruction of erythrocytes, and resultant haemolysis. *Haemolytic uraemic syndrome* (HUS) and *thrombotic thrombocytopenic purpura* (TTP) are two types of thrombotic microangiopathy. In HUS, renal vessels are mainly affected, whereas in TTP, systemic involvement, especially in the brain is predominant. Both conditions may cause renal failure. *Escherichia coli* O157-associated diarrhoea may cause HUS/TTP, and is now the main cause of acute renal failure in children in the UK. Note that thrombotic microangiopathy may progress into *disseminated intravascular coagulopathy* (DIC) – see chapter on bleeding tendency.

Structural disorders
Polycystic kidney disease
Polycystic kidney disease is characterized by the formation of multiple cysts in the renal parenchyma, leading to marked enlargement of the kidneys and progressive renal failure. Two types of polycystic kidney disease exist: infantile (autosomal recessive) and adult (autosomal dominant) polycystic kidney disease. Adult polycystic kidney disease is caused by defects in one of three genes, PKD1, PKD2 or PKD3.

Alport's syndrome
Alport's syndrome is an inherited disease caused by mutations in the gene for Type IV collagen in the basement membrane of the glomerulus. Progressive degeneration

of the glomerulus occurs, leading to glomerulonephritis. Other tissues may be affected by the mutation in collagen, e.g. deafness may result from cochlear dysfunction.

Investigations in renal failure

Renal failure is diagnosed by blood measurement of urea and electrolytes. Serum urea, creatinine and potassium, which are normally cleared by the kidney, may be raised, and metabolic acidosis causes the plasma bicarbonate to be low. Serial measurement of these markers is vital to monitoring the progress of renal failure and to prevent hyperkalaemia. Hyperkalaemia (serum potassium >6 mmol/L) is danger-ous, since it may lead to cardiac arrest if untreated. In CRF, serum calcium is typically low (due to osteomalacia) and phosphate is high (reduced renal clearance).

A 24-hour urine collection sent for *creatinine clearance* is useful to measure the severity of renal failure precisely. Urine microscopy should be performed, since the presence of *red cell casts* is suggestive of GN.

Ultrasound scan and *Doppler* imaging of the kidneys is important to exclude outflow obstruction of urine (i.e. post-renal failure). It is also useful to look at the structure and size of the kidneys, since in CRF the kidneys tend to become small and atrophic. The Doppler image gives an estimation of blood flow in the renal arteries, in order to screen for renal artery stenosis or renal vein thrombosis.

Immunological blood tests are performed to look for certain causes of GN:

- *ANCA*: pANCA is associated with polyarteritis nodosa. (It is also associated with inflammatory bowel disease and HIV infection.) cANCA is associated with Wegener's granulomatosis.
- *Anti-GBM antibody* is diagnostic of Goodpasture's syndrome.
- *Anti-nuclear antigen* (ANA) and double-stranded DNA (dsDNA) are associated with SLE.
- *Serum complement* (C3, C4): a low complement C3<<C4 is associated with SLE.

A *MAG-3 scan* is a specialist investigation used to measure the excretion of radioiso-tope from the blood into each kidney. It therefore allows assessment of the function of each kidney individually.

Renal biopsy is the gold standard method for diagnosing the type of renal failure. It is associated uncommonly with significant complications such as uncontrolled bleeding and worsening of renal failure.

Management of renal failure

There are five principles of management of renal failure.

Treatment of underlying disease

In primary glomerular disease this usually consists of immunosuppressive agents such as high-dose corticosteroids, with or without other agents such as azathioprine and cyclophosphamide.

Fluid balance

If oliguria or anuria is present, strict restriction of oral fluid intake is vital to prevent fluid overload (and thus pulmonary oedema). Haemodialysis may be needed if symptomatic fluid overload occurs.

Correction of biochemical abnormalities
Acute hyperkalaemia should be treated immediately with intravenous (IV) calcium gluconate and IV insulin with 50% dextrose. If renal failure is severe or persistent, hyperkalaemia (>6 mmol/L), acidosis and uraemia may all need to be corrected with dialysis.

Haemodialysis involves the circulation of blood through a machine where ions diffuse across a selectively permeable membrane into dialysate fluid. Blood is either drawn from the patient with a plastic venous catheter or via an arteriovenous fistula surgically formed in the arm, and is heparinised.

An alternative to haemodialysis is continuous ambulatory peritoneal dialysis (CAPD), which involves regular exchanges of dialysis fluid into the peritoneal cavity via a Tenckhoff catheter in the abdominal wall. CAPD may be complicated by peritonitis from infection of the Tenckhoff catheter.

Prevention and treatment of complications of CRF
See section on complications of CRF.

Transplantation
Transplantation of either a live-related or cadaveric kidney provides a cure for CRF, and has a 70–80% success rate after 5 years.

Urinary tract calculi

Urinary tract calculi (stones) consist principally of aggregates of crystals of various types. Calculi may occur anywhere in the renal tract, including the renal pelvis, ureter and bladder. Different types of calculus may be formed, but about 80% are calcium oxalate or phosphate. Magnesium/ammonium phosphate constitutes a further 10%. Urate and cysteine stones are rare.

Factors contributing to stone formation include:

- *Urinary stasis* caused by low urine volumes (e.g. in hot weather), which promote crystal formation.
- *Urinary tract infection.*
- *Increased urinary excretion of a salt.* Disorders such as renal tubular acidosis and vitamin D excess may lead to increased calcium salt deposition. Thiazide diuretics and gout lead to increased urate formation and excretion. Inherited enzyme defects such as cystinuria and primary oxaluria also lead to stone formation.

Colicky severe loin pain (*renal colic*) which radiates into the groin is characteristic. Urinary frequency, dysuria and microscopic haematuria also occur. Stones promote urinary tract infection, and may cause acute or chronic urinary tract obstruction (and thus post-renal failure).

About 90% of renal stones are visible on a plain abdominal X-ray. An intravenous urogram (IVU) will show delayed filling and dilatation of the obstructed ureter with radio-opaque contrast; however, spiral computed tomography (CT) is increasingly used to detect calculi.

Renal colic should be treated with strong analgesia (either diclofenac, pethidine or morphine). Most small stones (under 4 mm) will pass spontaneously with adequate oral fluid intake (at least 2 litres per day). For other stones, extracorporeal shock wave lithotripsy (ESWL) is a non-invasive technique used to break the stones into smaller pieces which may pass out in the urine. Alternatively, cystoscopy, or even open surgery may be required to remove stones.

Renal neoplasms

Renal cell carcinoma

The most common renal neoplasm in adults is renal cell carcinoma (RCC), a malignant neoplasm arising from renal tubular cells. It is more common in men, and has a peak incidence in middle-aged people. Smoking is a risk factor for its development, and there is an inherited form of bilateral RCC which appears as part of von Hippel–Lindau syndrome.

The classical clinical triad of symptoms for RCC is loin pain, abdominal mass and haematuria; however, all three features present together only rarely. RCC has a predilection for direct, continuous spread along the renal vein to the inferior vena cava. Other features include pyrexia, polycythaemia (due to ectopic erythropoietin production) and hypertension (due to renin production). RCC may be diagnosed with renal ultrasound or contrast-enhanced CT. Radical nephrectomy is often curative if the tumour has no distal spread, but with metastatic disease, response to chemotherapy and radiotherapy is poor. Immunotherapy with interleukin-2 can be helpful, but overall survival is poor in metastatic disease.

Transitional cell carcinoma

Transitional cell carcinoma (TCC) is a malignant neoplasm of the uroepithelium which most commonly occurs in the bladder, but may also appear in the ureter or renal pelvis. Risk factors include smoking and exposure to certain carcinogens used in chemical and dye factories.

TCC most commonly presents with asymptomatic haematuria, but may also cause loin pain. Investigation with urine cytology may reveal malignant cells. If IVU (to examine the whole urinary tract) or retrograde ureteropyelogram (to look at the ureters and renal pelvises) demonstrate a suspicious lesion, further investigation with cystoscopy or ureteroscopy with biopsy is then needed to make the diagnosis.

Treatment of renal TCC is usually nephrectomy. Bladder tumours are treated with surgery (local excision or cystectomy), radiotherapy and/or chemotherapy (local or systemic), depending on the stage and grade of the tumour.

Dental aspects of renal disease

Careful haemostasis should be ensured if oral surgical procedures are necessary.

Drugs which are directly nephrotoxic must be avoided and drugs excreted mainly by the kidney may have undesirably enhanced or prolonged activity if doses are not lowered.

Infections are poorly controlled in CRF, especially if the patient is immunosuppressed, and may spread locally as well as giving rise to septicaemia. Odontogenic infections should be treated vigorously.

Consideration for antimicrobial prophylaxis before extractions, scaling or periodontal surgery includes:

- Patients with polycystic kidneys (who may also have mitral valve prolapse).
- Patients receiving peritoneal dialysis, since bacteraemia can result in peritonitis in those on CAPD or CCPD (continuous cyclic peritoneal dialysis).
- Some patients on haemodialysis. Vascular access infections are usually caused by skin organisms such as *Staphylococcus aureus* and only rarely by oral microorganisms. Patients with most arteriovenous fistulas are therefore not considered at risk from infection during dental treatment. However, those with prosthetic bridge grafts of polytetrafluoroethylene or tunnelled cuffed catheters may need to be managed with precautions similar to those at risk from infective endocarditis (see chapter on infective endocarditis).
- Patients with transplants (see chapter on transplantation).

Osseous lesions include loss of the lamina dura, osteoporosis and osteolytic areas (renal osteodystrophy). Secondary hyperparathyroidism may lead to giant cell lesions.

Five facts

1. By far the most common cause (80%) of renal failure is inadequate renal perfusion (pre-renal failure), e.g. due to dehydration, hypotension or sepsis.
2. Post-renal failure is the second-most common cause of renal failure, and may be caused by obstruction anywhere in the renal tract.
3. The most important immediate danger in renal failure is hyperkalaemia (>6 mmol/L), which may lead to cardiac arrest.
4. People with renal failure may be oliguric, which puts them at high risk of becoming fluid overloaded and developing pulmonary oedema.
5. Renal patients have increased bleeding, increased risk of infection and prolonged wound healing.

Sexually transmitted diseases

Sexually transmitted diseases (STDs) are, by definition, diseases which are primarily transmitted via sexual contact. They were previously known as venereal diseases. Intimate contact is required for their transmission – they are not as highly contagious as, for example, airborne infections such as respiratory viruses.

The high profile of diseases such as HIV/AIDS has led to a huge effort to promote preventative measures such as sex education, contraception and improved access to genitourinary medicine (GUM) clinics.

The main STDs are shown in Table 1, but most common of these are chlamydia, herpes, human papillomavirus infections and gonorrhoea. The incidence of all STDs are increasing currently, mainly because of sexual promiscuity.

The risk of infections with STDs can be reduced by avoiding casual and unprotected sexual intercourse by ABC:

- Abstinence
- Being monogamous
- Condom use always.

Table 1 The major STDs together with their causative organisms

Disease	Causal microorganisms
Chlamydial infections	*Chlamydia trachomatis*
Gonorrhoea	*Neisseria gonorrhoeae*
Hepatitis B	Hepatitis B virus
Herpes	Herpes simplex virus
HIV/AIDS	Human immunodeficiency virus
Syphilis	*Treponema pallidum*
Trichomoniasis	*Trichomonas vaginalis*
Warts	Human papillomaviruses

Three important principles should be used when managing STDs:

1. Although confidentiality and sensitivity are important when dealing with any medical condition, they are absolutely vital with STDs.
2. An individual with one STD is at high risk of having another STD. Individuals should therefore be tested for other common STDs.
3. Contact tracing – sexual partners (past and present) need to be traced so that they may be offered testing and treatment.

Chlamydia

Chlamydia trachomatis is an intracellular bacterium that accounts for about half of cases of non-gonococcal urethritis (see below), and is also associated with Reiter's syndrome (see below).

Clinical features

Common clinical features of chlamydial infection include urethritis, cervicitis, vaginal bleeding, pelvic inflammatory disease (PID) and conjunctivitis, but most females remain asymptomatic. Chlamydia can be spread during childbirth to the baby, causing ophthalmia neonatorum (conjunctivitis) or pneumonia.

Reiter's syndrome

Reiter's syndrome is defined clinically as a triad of:

1. conjunctivitis
2. arthritis
3. urethritis.

Reiter's syndrome is HLA-B27 associated, and is caused by either chlamydia-associated urethritis, or colitis caused by *Salmonella, Shigella* or *Yersinia*. Oral red patches may be seen.

Non-gonococcal urethritis in males

Typical features of this disease include dysuria and urethral discharge. It is defined as the presence of >5 polymorphs on high-power (×1000) microscopy. *Chlamydia* accounts for about half the cases. Other causes include:

- *Ureaplasma urealyticum*
- *Mycoplasma genitalium*
- *Candida albicans*
- *Neisseria meningitidis.*

Investigations

Chlamydia may be seen as intracellular inclusion bodies using immunofluorescence. It may be grown in cell or chick embryo culture.

Management

Doxycycline or azithromycin are both effective in curing infection in the majority of cases.

Gonorrhoea

Gonorrhoea is caused by infection with the Gram-negative diplococcus *Neisseria gonorrhoeae.*

Clinical features

Urethritis may cause dysuria and purulent urethral discharge. *Proctitis* (inflammation of the rectum) may occur after infection due to anal sex. *Cervicitis* may produce vaginal discharge and pelvic pain. *Conjunctivitis* causes inflammation with a purulent discharge from the eyes.

Pelvic inflammatory disease is a late complication of infection of the female reproductive tract. Inflammation leads to chronic pelvic pain, dyspareunia (pain during sexual intercourse) and may result in infertility.

Note that about 50% of women with gonorrhoea are asymptomatic, and gonorrhoeal proctitis is often undiagnosed.

Investigations
Microscopy and culture of any infected fluid will confirm the diagnosis.

Management
Ciprofloxacin (a fluoroquinolone) is the first-line agent used to treat gonorrhoea.

Dental aspects
The oropharynx seems to be infrequently affected, except perhaps in male homosexuals.

Herpes simplex

See chapter on dermatological conditions.

Hepatitis B and C

See chapter on liver disease.

HIV

See chapter on HIV and AIDS.

HPV (ano-genital warts)

See chapter on dermatological conditions.

Syphilis

Syphilis is caused by infection with the spirochaete *Treponema pallidum*. The incidence of syphilis has continued to rise in recent years, with epidemics in some cities, especially among men who engage in homosexual intercourse.

Clinical features
Syphilis infection may be divided into primary, secondary, latent and tertiary infection. Furthermore, congenital syphilis may occur.

Primary syphilis (2–4 weeks after infection)
- *Chancre* – a red macule forms at the site of infection, typically in the ano-genital region, e.g. glans penis, vulva. This develops into a papule, which ulcerates to form a *chancre*. The chancre, which is pale and painless, spontaneously heals after about a month.
- *Inguinal lymphadenopathy* may be present.

Secondary syphilis (2 months after infection)
- *Maculopapular rash* – asymptomatic, and involves the trunk and limbs, including the palms and soles.
- *Condylomata lata* – papules forming plaques may be present in the genital areas.
- *Generalized lymphadenopathy* is often present.
- *Constitutional symptoms* such as tiredness and a fever may be present.

Latent phase
Without treatment, syphilis may remain asymptomatic for many years or even the rest of the individual's life. For the first 2 years, individuals are still infectious. However, subsequently, they can only transmit infection vertically to the fetus.

Tertiary syphilis (3–10 years after infection)
Chronic granulomatous lesions referred to as gummata (singular = gumma) form in multiple organs.

- *Skin*: gummata may form ulcers or nodules, which heal with scarring. If they are subcutaneous, gum-like material may discharge to the skin surface.
- *Mucosa of mouth, nose, pharynx*: gummata appear as punched-out ulcers.
- *Cardiovascular*: aortic incompetence and aortitis with formation of thoracic aortic aneurysm may occur.
- *Neurological*: meningitis, tabes dorsalis and generalized paresis of the insane are all clinical syndromes produced by syphilitic infection.

Congenital syphilis
Congenital infection may cause spontaneous abortion of the fetus. If the fetus survives, congenital syphilis may produce characteristic clinical features in the neonatal period or later in childhood. Such features include:

- facies – saddle nose, maxillary hypoplasia, Hutchinson's (screw-driver shaped) incisors, high arched palate
- bones – periostitis
- hepatosplenomegaly – in neonates
- features of secondary or tertiary syphilis.

Investigation
Serology
VDRL (Venereal Disease Research Laboratory) provides a non-specific but useful screening test. However, it may give false-positive results, e.g. in antiphospholipid syndrome and infectious mononucleosis. TPHA (*T. pallidum* haemagglutination assay) and FTA-ABS (fluorescent treponemal antibody absorption test) are two specific tests for syphilis.

Microscopy
Fluid from chancres or gummata may be examined under dark-field microscopy for *T. pallidum* organisms. CSF (cerebrospinal fluid) may also reveal organisms in tertiary syphilis.

Treatment
Early identification and treatment with penicillin is the treatment of choice.

Dental aspects
Primary chancres occasionally involve the lips or tongue. Painless oral ulcers (mucous patches and snailtrack ulcers) classically appear in the second stage but are seen in only about one-third of patients. The main oral manifestation of tertiary syphilis is leukoplakia, particularly of the dorsum of the tongue, which has a high potential for malignant change. Mucosal gummata may destroy bone, particularly the palate, or involve the tongue.

Five facts

1. STDs are increasing in frequency due to sexual promiscuity.
2. Syphilis, herpes simplex and (uncommonly) gonorrhoea are associated with oral lesions.
3. An individual with an STD should be screened for other STDs due to their increased risk.
4. Partners (past and present) of individuals with an STD must be screened as well.
5. With the exception of herpes simplex and warts, STDs are *not* transmissible via direct contact with skin or mucosal surfaces.

Shock and haemorrhage

Types of shock

Shock is defined as a state in which tissue perfusion and oxygenation are inadequate to maintain organ function. The basic cause is that not enough well-oxygenated blood is getting to the tissues and this can be due to:

- Respiratory failure – where the tissues receive enough blood but the blood is not well-oxygenated.
- Circulatory failure – which can be either (a) pump (cardiogenic) failure due to cardiac muscle failure, arrhythmias, valve disease, obstruction from pulmonary embolus, pulmonary valve stenosis or coronary heart disease, or (b) a lack of circulating volume (hypovolaemia) due to blood loss, fluid loss (e.g. burns), intestinal obstruction or peritonitis, or (c) fluid maldistribution such as in sepsis or anaphylaxis.

Classification

Shock can therefore be hypovolaemic, cardiogenic, neurogenic (sympathetic nervous system failure), septic or anaphylactic.

Pathophysiology

The impaired tissue perfusion and resultant ischaemia are associated with anaerobic metabolism and generalized cellular damage. These result in the formation of lactic acid and a consequent metabolic acidosis, which is best assessed using arterial blood gases (ABG). Furthermore, the switch from aerobic to anaerobic metabolism means that much less ATP is formed, and thus the cellular Na/K pump fails. This then causes Na and H_2O influx into cells, which then swell and pull away from each other, allowing fluid to escape into the interstitium and disrupt the integrity of the individual organs.

If this process continues, multiple organ dysfunction syndrome (MODS) can result, which if untreated can become irreversible – multiple organ failure (MOF) – with a high mortality (50% if two organs have failed, 80% if three organs). Hence it is vital to try and prevent this cascade.

Haemorrhage

Haemorrhage is the commonest cause of shock and leads to loss of circulating blood and fluid (hypovolaemic shock). It should always be suspected in any case of haemodynamic compromise due to major trauma, although it can coexist with other causes (e.g. cardiogenic with chest trauma, septic with infection, and neurogenic with spinal trauma).

Severe haemorrhage may not always be easy to recognize. Possible locations of such 'hidden haemorrhage' are in the thorax, abdomen (especially the retroperitoneal space), pelvic fractures or from blood spilt at the site of injury: i.e. 'in the chest, in the belly or on the road'.

Diagnosis

The clinical features of shock can be worked out if the student has a basic grasp of the relevant cardiac physiology:

Cardiac output (CO) = Stroke volume (SV) × Heart rate (HR)

Blood pressure (BP) = Cardiac output (CO) × Peripheral vascular resistance (PVR)

With the tissues not receiving enough well-oxygenated blood, the body tries to compensate by increasing CO. This it does by increasing the HR; thus, *an early sign of shock is tachycardia*. The body also tries to maintain BP so that oxygen can get to the tissues, and therefore the sympathetic nervous system is activated to produce peripheral vasoconstriction, and increase the PVR, thus maintaining BP until the later stages of shock. This vasoconstriction leads to *cold, clammy peripheries, and the patient looking dehydrated ('peripheral shutdown')*.

The patient also tries to compensate by increasing oxygenation; therefore *the respiratory rate increases*. The kidneys shut down the production of urine in an attempt to maintain circulating volume, but this is a late sign. The lack of blood flow to the brain as shock increases causes deterioration in the mental state as a late sign.

Other types of shock may have slightly different features; for example, in neurogenic shock the sympathetic failure means that there is no tachycardia, and in septic shock the peripheries are warm due to the inflammatory response.

Management

Maintaining oxygen delivery is the key to improving survival. Early aggressive management is often the only chance to prevent mortality and it is imperative that specialist medical advice is sought in any patient suspected to be in shock.

The aim of treatment is resuscitation – airway, breathing and circulation (ABC) as detailed in the chapter on trauma and advanced trauma life support (ATLS). This allows maximal oxygen delivery to the tissues. 'A' and 'B' are maintained with adequate ventilatory support and oxygenation. 'C,' which is compromised in haemorrhagic shock, is managed by controlling any obvious sources of bleeding with direct pressure and elevation, fluid replacement and cardiac support.

Fluid can be replaced intravenously after the insertion of two large-bore (grey/brown) cannulae into large peripheral (e.g. antecubital fossa) veins. If initial access is difficult, a cutdown on to the great saphenous vein can be performed by someone experienced with this procedure (not the dentist!). In children under 8 years of age, it is often quicker to insert an intraosseus cannula into the femur or tibia but this should only be done by those with Advanced Paediatric Life Support (APLS) training. Once access has been obtained, fluid can be run in as quickly as possible initially and then titrated to the patient's clinical response.

The question of what replacement fluid to use is a matter of debate. Crystalloids are fluids that do not contain proteins, and colloids are those that do. Colloids therefore are more 'physiological', i.e. more like the plasma that the patient has lost and thus in theory might seem more attractive to use. However, they do not remain in the circulation as long as crystalloids and are more likely to cause an anaphylactoid reaction. ATLS teaching states that fluid resuscitation should begin with colloid to increase the circulating volume rapidly and then move on to crystalloids to maintain it. Typically, in resuscitation, Hartmann's solution (known as Ringer's lactate in the USA) is the colloid of choice (although occasionally Gelofusine or Haemaccel are used), and the crystalloid of choice is isotonic (also called normal) saline (0.9%).

In severe haemorrhage, blood transfusion may be needed, and therefore at the time of intravenous (IV) cannulation it is important to send blood for cross-match (as well as for assay of haemoglobin, glucose, renal function, etc.). It takes about 1 hour to get fully cross-matched blood available; in an emergency type-specific (takes 10 min to prepare) or type O blood (universal donor as it has no antigens and thus can be given to anyone) is used instead. It is important to remember that if not fully cross-matched, rhesus negative blood must be used in females of childbearing age.

Whatever type of fluid resuscitation is employed, the fluid should be warmed towards body temperature before infusion so as to avoid making the patient hypothermic. Autotransfusion – whereby the lost blood is collected and infused back into the patient – is theoretically possible in clean trauma, but is uncommon in practice.

Cardiac support to improve pump function may also be required in shock as not only does the blood need to be well-oxygenated but it also needs to be pumped to the tissues. This is ensured by the maintenance of a good CO, by increasing SV or HR. Drugs that increase SV are inotropes and those that increase HR are chronotropes. Such agents should only be used in a specialist setting such as the intensive treatment unit (ITU) by doctors trained in their use.

To help with monitoring the response to cardiac drugs and fluid resuscitation, the patient may have a central venous pressure (CVP) line inserted, typically into one of the internal jugular or subclavian veins. This then allows monitoring of the pressure inside the right atrium of the heart, which is an indirect measure of left ventricular pressure and therefore the volume status of the patient. Further fluid resuscitation and cardiac support can then be tailored to the CVP and clinical state of the patient.

It is important to be aware that certain conditions make the CVP an unreliable indicator of volume status (e.g. myocardial infarction, tension pneumothorax, air embolism, cardiac contusion, pericardial effusion).

Monitoring

Regular monitoring is essential in shocked patients so that treatment can be constantly titrated to response. The HR, BP, respiratory rate, urine output, temperature, conscious level, CVP, blood tests and ABG should be regularly assessed. Once stabilized, the patient may require transfer to a higher level of care where such monitoring is readily available.

Complications

Complications which are serious and require specialist medical or ITU management include:

- MODS
- MOF
- acute renal failure
- acute respiratory distress syndrome
- gastrointestinal stress ulceration
- disseminated intravascular coagulation.

Prognosis

The prognosis depends on the underlying cause, severity and duration of the shock and the efficacy of treatment. Increasing age and co-morbidity decrease survival.

Dental aspects

Shock is most likely to be encountered in trauma patients, who may also have maxillo-facial injuries.

Five facts

1. Shock is a state of inadequate tissue perfusion.
2. Hypovolaemic shock is most commonly due to haemorrhage, commonly from trauma.
3. Tachycardia is an early sign of shock; hypotension is a late sign.
4. ABC principles are paramount in management.
5. Multi-organ failure is a serious complication of shock that has a high mortality.

Stroke

A stroke is the syndrome of rapidly developing disturbance of cerebral function lasting >24 hours, or death within that time. Strokes may be preceded by transient ischaemic attacks (TIA), which are typically embolic, and may cause focal cerebral deficits usually lasting <60 min and recovering fully within 24 hours. A reversible ischaemic neurological deficit (RIND) is similar but persists for >24 hours.

Epidemiology

Strokes are a common cause of death and disability, especially in the elderly. They are the third leading cause of death, account for 1 out of every 15 deaths in the developed world, and are the leading cause of disability in adults. Stroke is common, with an incidence of approximately 2 per 1000 people per year. Men are affected twice as often as women and the incidence doubles with each decade after age 35. Strokes affect around 5% of men aged 65–74 years old, and 12% of those older.

Classification

Stroke may be caused by three completely distinct pathological processes:

*   cerebral infarction   85% of strokes
*   subarachnoid haemorrhage   10% of strokes
*   intracerebral haemorrhage   5% of strokes.

Cerebral infarction

The majority of strokes are caused by interruption of the blood supply to one of the cerebral arteries. Cerebral infarction is mostly caused by arterial thrombosis, but may also occur secondary to embolism.

Cerebral arterial thrombosis is the most common cause of stroke, follows atherosclerosis and tends to be the least rapid in its development; it has a lower acute mortality (30%).

Cerebral emboli may originate from an atherosclerotic carotid artery or arch of aorta. They may also arise from *in situ* thrombus in the heart, especially in atrial fibrillation or post-myocardial infarction.

Pathogenesis

After occlusion of the cerebral artery (whether via thrombosis or embolism), ischaemia, and eventually infarction, occurs. The mechanism of infarction involves the release of glutamate (a neurotransmitter) from damaged cells, which cause influx of calcium; this process is called *excitotoxicity*.

Risk factors for cerebral infarction include smoking, hypertension, previous TIA or stroke, diabetes, hyperlipidaemia, heart disease, sex steroids and cocaine use.

Clinical features
Strokes caused by cerebral infarction are clinically classified according to the time course of resolution and/or worsening of deficits.

Transient ischaemic attacks
Transient ischaemic attacks are typically embolic and may cause focal cerebral deficits such as facial numbness, hemiplegia or dysarthria, usually lasting <60 min and recovering fully within 24 hours. About 30% of TIAs progress to strokes.

Reversible ischaemic neurological deficit
A RIND is similar to a TIA but persists for >24 hours.

Stroke-in-evolution
A stroke-in-evolution is when such a deficit persists and worsens. Common features include changes in vision, speech and comprehension; weakness; vertigo; loss of sensation in a part of the body; or changes in the level of consciousness.

Full stroke
A full stroke causes deficits which persist but do not worsen. Over days and weeks, the deficits may partially resolve. Typical features of a complete stroke include:

* hemiplegia (loss of voluntary movement of the opposite side of the body to the lesion)

Table 1 Clinical features of stroke caused by occlusion of individual cerebral arteries

Artery occluded	Clinical features	Area of brain damaged
Middle cerebral artery	*Contralateral hemiplegia*: weakness of opposite side of body (mainly leg)	Motor cortex (parietal lobe)
	Dysphagia (difficulty swallowing)	Motor cortex
	Dysarthria (difficulty articulating words)	Motor cortex
	Dysphasia (difficulty either expressing or understanding speech)	Broca's (expression) and Wernicke's (understanding) area
Posterior cerebral artery	Visual field deficits	Visual cortex (occipital lobe)
Vertebral or basilar arteries	Autonomic disturbances	Brainstem
	Impaired consciousness	
	Motor, cranial nerve, sensory deficits	
Anterior cerebral arteries	Contralateral hemiplegia: mainly face and arm	Frontal lobes
Deep penetrating arteries	Purely motor, purely sensory, sensory and motor	Internal capsule (this is a *lacunar* infarct)
	Visual field defects	

- loss of speech (aphasia)
- loss of or deterioration in vision.

There is a high mortality from strokes, related not only to the acute brain damage but also to complications such as thrombosis and infection, especially respiratory. Stroke-related symptoms depend on the area of brain affected, the extent of damage and the cause, but may include a wide range of clinical syndromes depending on the artery occluded, and therefore the area of brain which infarcts (Table 1).

Subarachnoid haemorrhage

Subarachnoid haemorrhage (SAH), which accounts for about 10% of strokes, originates from the rupture of a congenital aneurysm (berry aneurysm) of the arterial circle of Willis, and since blood can burst through the brain into a cerebral ventricle, death may follow within a few minutes. Blood enters the subarachnoid space, causing sudden onset of meningeal irritation. The prognosis of SAH is poor and about 30% of patients die from the initial haemorrhage. Only 50% survive the stroke.

Meningeal irritation causes photophobia, neck stiffness and a severe, occipital headache of sudden onset. The headache is often described as 'being hit over the back of the head with a baseball bat'.

Risk factors for the formation of berry aneurysms include hypertension and connective tissue disorders.

Intracerebral haemorrhage

Intracerebral haemorrhage, which mainly affects those beyond middle age, is the most lethal type of stroke, with a mortality of 80%, since bleeding into the brain destroys and tears apart the tissue.

Intracerebral haemorrhage results from the rupture of Charcot–Bouchard microaneurysms, which form in the brain parenchyma as a result of hypertension. They cause a rapid rise in intracranial pressure, but may also cause focal neurological deficits corresponding to the area of brain parenchyma damaged.

Intracerebral haemorrhage presents with sudden onset of features of raised intracranial pressure, such as impaired consciousness, nausea/vomiting and headache. Focal neurological deficits may also be seen.

Acute investigation and management of stroke

The airway must be protected during the acute phase in patients with a reduced level of consciousness. For virtually all strokes, hospitalization is required, possibly including intensive care and life support. Oxygen is given to all patients as is typical of most emergencies.

- *Aspirin* has been shown to improve survival in cerebral infarction if given early.
- *Keep the patient 'nil by mouth' until a swallow assessment is done* to prevent risk of aspiration.
- *Computed tomography (CT) scan of head* is performed urgently if haemorrhagic stroke is suspected. Note that infarcts will not show up on CT scans within 24 hours.

- *Lumbar puncture* is performed if SAH is suspected but CT scan is normal. Blood and haemosiderin in the cerebrospinal fluid indicates a bleed.
- *Neurosurgery* – patients with haemorrhagic stroke should be urgently referred to a neurosurgical team. Treatment with nimodipine to reduce intracranial vasospasm, and neurosurgery to clip the aneurysm in SAH can be curative. In some other cases, surgical removal of blood clots from the brain may be indicated.

Chronic investigation and management of stroke

- *Carotid dopplers* are used to look for stenosis of carotid arteries from atherosclerosis. Severely stenosed arteries may be treated with surgery to remove atherosclerotic plaques from them, but this itself has a stroke complication rate of 5% and a mortality rate of 1–2%.
- *Echocardiography* is done to look for thrombus in the heart chambers. If thrombus is seen, warfarin anticoagulation may be initiated.
- *Serum glucose and lipids* are tested to screen for diabetes and hyperlipidaemia.
- *Screening and reduction of risk factors* such as hypertension and atrial fibrillation (AF) is vital in preventing further strokes. Anticoagulation with warfarin for AF may be intitiated 10 days after the stroke if it is certain that the stroke is thrombotic or embolic.
- *Rehabilitation in a stroke unit* significantly improves morbidity and mortality by preventing complications (e.g. bed sores and limb contractures), and provides good access to physiotherapy, speech therapy and occupational therapy.

Main dental aspects

Since a person who has had a TIA, RIND or stroke is at greater risk of another, elective dental care should be deferred for 6 months. Dental management modifications in a patient with a stroke may also include consideration of problems of access and impaired mobility, communication and loss of protective reflexes.

It is thus important to have short stress-free treatment sessions in the mid morning, monitor BP and use a minimal amount of adrenaline (epinephrine) in local anaesthesia. Calcified atherosclerotic plaques may sometimes be detected on dental panoramic radiographs.

Five facts

1. Most strokes (85%) are caused by cerebral infarction (either due to in situ thrombosis or embolism).
2. Haemorrhagic strokes (15% of all strokes) may be due to a subarachnoid haemorrhage or intracerebral bleed.
3. The neurological features of a stroke are highly variable, depending on the type of stroke and the area of the brain affected.
4. Haemorrhagic strokes must be urgently referred to a neurosurgical team.
5. Dental considerations with stroke patients include problems with impaired mobility, communication and loss of protective reflexes, e.g. cough reflex.

Thromboembolic disease

Thromboembolic disease is the third commonest cause of death in hospitalized patients in the UK, usually arising as thrombosis in a deep leg vein (deep vein thrombosis; DVT), which detaches and comes to rest in the pulmonary artery (pulmonary embolism). This occurs especially postoperatively and can also be seen in air travel (economy class syndrome).

Predisposition to venous thrombosis in the leg and pelvic veins after surgery arises from three components (the so-called Virchow's triad):

1. Increased thrombotic tendency – after blood loss and platelet consumption intraoperatively, more platelets are produced and they have an increased tendency to aggregate. Fibrinogen levels also increase postoperatively.
2. Changes in blood flow – immobilization on the operating table and in bed postoperatively causes stagnation of venous blood flow.
3. Damage to the vein wall – pressure of the operating table and direct damage to vein endothelia intraoperatively allow thrombus formation on the damaged vein segment.

Patients undergoing major surgery, especially on the lower limbs and/or pelvis, are especially at risk of DVT. Other risk factors include:

- elderly
- malignancy
- obesity
- varicose veins
- previous history of deep vein thrombosis
- oral contraceptive pill (OCP) use
- hormone replacement therapy (HRT) use
- protein C/S deficiency
- factor V Leiden mutation.

Deep vein thrombosis (DVT)

DVT can be 'silent' (i.e. asymptomatic) or can present with calf pain – typically in the second postoperative week. On examination the calf is hot, swollen and tender, and the pain is worsened by ankle plantarflexion (Homan's sign). The patient is usually also systemically unwell and pyrexial. If the pelvic or femoral veins are affected, then the poor venous drainage causes swelling of the whole lower limb.

D-dimers are breakdown products of fibrinogen (also called fibrinogen breakdown products, FBPs) that are classically produced in patients with DVT and can be detected in the blood. However, since fibrinogen is normally broken down after surgery, this simple blood test is of no use in the diagnosis of postoperative patients. Doppler ultrasound scanning is a simple, non-invasive, reliable method of diagnosing DVT in veins above the knee. For calf and smaller DVT it is difficult to visualize thrombi using Doppler, even with duplex techniques. However, the significance of below-knee DVT, thought to be present in >70% of postoperative patients, is controversial. Although venography is cited by many textbooks to be the gold standard investigation, it is seldom used in clinical practice due to its invasive nature.

Prophylactic measures

Given the potentially preventable nature of DVT, several prophylactic measures should be instituted.

In all *surgical patients*, precautions include:

- The oral contraceptive should be stopped several weeks preoperatively, and other risk factors should be minimized if at all possible.
- Intraoperatively, intermittent pneumatic calf compression and head-down tilt is used by some surgeons to stimulate blood flow.
- Early mobilization to stimulate blood flow should be encouraged in the postoperative period.
- Thromboembolic disease (TED) stockings cause graded compression from heel to knee, and will aid venous blood flow up the leg and help prevent stagnation.

In *high-risk patients*, subcutaneous injections of low molecular weight heparin (e.g. enoxaparin) should also be started preoperatively and continued while the patient remains at risk. The use of heparin agents has been shown in numerous studies to reduce the incidence of DVT, and subsequent pulmonary embolism. Continuous intravenous heparin administration, which necessitates regular blood tests (activated partial thromboplastin time or APTT) to check correct dosage, is now unpopular. All hospital admissions, both acute and elective, should be assessed for thromboembolic risk, although a recent audit by the first author (P.S.)[1] showed that much improvement is needed by medical staff in this area.

Management of DVT

In patients already diagnosed with DVT, the crucial point is to reduce the risk of embolization, particularly pulmonary embolization. Anticoagulant therapy with heparin (either intravenously or subcutaneously) will both help prevent further clot propagation and increase fibrinolysis. Once fully anticoagulated, heparin therapy is replaced with oral warfarin treatment. It is important to remember that in the immediate postoperative period anticoagulant therapy may increase the risk of significant haemorrhage, and should therefore not be instituted without senior surgical advice. If bleeding does occur in treated patients, then protamine sulphate can be used to reverse the heparin effect.

Pulmonary embolus (PE)

Classically, PE occurs around day 10 postoperatively. The size of the pulmonary arterial vessel that is blocked by the PE will determine the severity of the condition, which can thus vary from mild symptoms of dyspnoea (shortness of breath) and mild pleuritic chest pain to sudden death from an occluded main pulmonary artery. Coughing up blood (haemoptysis) is a frequent symptom, as is confusion due to hypoxia in elderly patients. Cyanosis, obstructive shock and right heart failure are all poor prognostic signs and demand immediate management to prevent mortality.

PE can occur without any obvious DVT being found and, as both myocardial infarction and chest infection can mimic its presentation, a very high index of suspicion is needed to make the diagnosis. *Any postoperative patient who appears unwell, confused or recovering slower than expected should have this diagnosis considered.*

Many students forget that the lungs have a dual blood supply via the pulmonary and bronchial arteries and, therefore, if the pulmonary clot can be cleared, infarction of the lung is unlikely. However, repeated episodes of PE can cause pulmonary hypertension, making infarction more likely.

Diagnosis is confirmed by a ventilation/perfusion (V/Q) scan showing perfusion defects but normal ventilation. Chest radiography, which may show wedge shadowing, is unreliable. Electrocardiography (ECG) shows the classical pattern of right heart strain or 'S1 Q3 T3' (S wave in lead 1, and Q wave and inverted T wave in lead 3) in <25% cases. Arterial blood gases confirm hypoxia, but again are not diagnostic. Pulmonary angiography is the gold standard but is invasive.

PE is managed with oxygen, heparin anticoagulation and analgesia for the pain. Thrombolysis of large emboli using streptokinase or tissue plasminogen activator may be attempted via a pulmonary catheter. In extreme circumstances, thromboembolectomy with cardiopulmonary bypass may be considered by a cardiothoracic surgeon.

Recurrent PEs in well-anticoagulated patients may be prevented by insertion into the inferior vena cava (IVC) of a Greenfield filter – an umbrella-like device that catches emboli and stops their further progress up the venous tree.

Disseminated intravascular coagulation

Disseminated intravascular coagulation (DIC; consumption coagulopathy or defibrination syndrome) is an uncommon, complex and not fully understood process with potentially fatal activation of the haemostasis-related mechanisms within the circulation. It can lead to bleeding, thrombosis, haemolysis and shock. Precipitating causes include incompatible blood transfusions, severe sepsis, obstetric complications, burns and cancers in various sites or severe trauma.

DIC is an acute emergency; heparinization, replacement of clotting factors and platelets, or antifibrinolytic therapy must be given as appropriate.

Dental aspects

- In one series of head injuries, some degree of DIC was found in 57% of cases.
- Thrombophilia and hypofibrinolysis may possibly underlie so-called neuralgia-inducing cavitational osteonecrosis (NICO), which may cause severe jaw pain.

Reference

1. Sooriakumaran P, Burton L, Choudhary R et al. Are we good at thromboembolic disease prophylaxis? – an audit of the use of risk assessment forms. *Int J Clin Pract* (2005) in press.

Five facts

1. Venous thromboembolism (VTE) is the third commonest cause of death in hospitalized patients in the UK.
2. VTE is predisposed to by an increased thrombotic tendency, stagnation of blood flow and damage to the vessel wall (Virchow's triad).
3. Heparin and other anticoagulants are used for VTE prophylaxis in high-risk patients, including those undergoing major surgery.
4. The diagnosis of pulmonary embolus should be considered in any postoperative patient who appears unwell, confused or is recovering slower than expected.
5. DIC is associated with head injury and is an acute emergency requiring haematological input.

Thyroid disorders

Thyroid physiology

The thyroid gland synthesizes thyroxine (tetra-iodo-thyronine, T4) and tri-iodo-thyronine (T3)-iodine-containing hormones which control metabolic rate. T4 is converted to T3 in the periphery of the body and T3 is the active hormone.

Iodine in the diet is absorbed into the bloodstream as iodide, and taken up by the thyroid gland, where it is converted to organic iodine and bound to tyrosine radicals from thyroglobulin to form the thyroid hormones. Once released into the bloodstream, 99% of T3 and T4 circulate bound to protein. It is the small amount of 'free' thyroid hormones that produces the endocrine effects of the thyroid gland.

The immediate control of secretion of T3 and T4 is by thyroid-stimulating hormone (TSH) from the anterior pituitary gland. TSH is produced in response to low levels of T3 and T4 in the blood via a negative feedback mechanism, as is common in many endocrine loops. TSH is also released in response to hypothalamic thyrotrophin-releasing hormone (TRH).

Calcitonin is also secreted by the thyroid and works as an antagonist to the effects of parathyroid hormone (parathormone) by reducing serum calcium.

Goitres

A goitre is an enlargement of the thyroid gland, usually caused by excess stimulation by TSH. Excess TSH stimulation may be due to low levels of circulating thyroid hormones, or may be pathological (as in Graves' disease, see below). Physiological states that increase thyroid activity, such as pregnancy and puberty, are also associated with thyroid enlargement. These goitres are all termed 'simple hyperplastic' or 'colloid' goitres, and are not usually associated with clinical hyper- or hypo-function of the thyroid.

Occasionally, long-standing colloid goitres can become nodular goitres and then go on to cause thyroid dysfunction. Multinodular goitres develop in glands subjected to prolonged stimulation by TSH. They can therefore be endemic (in iodine-deficient areas) or sporadic (occurring haphazardly). These goitres are nodular, due to a disorganized response of the gland to stimulation, and contain areas of both hyperplasia and hypoplasia. When the nodules are hyperplastic, the patient may become hyperthyroid. In most long-standing nodular goitres though, the nodules are hypoplastic and the patient develops hypothyroidism. Sudden pain and enlargement can occur if there is haemorrhage into a nodule.

Solitary nodular goitres are less common than multinodular goitres. Indeed, in 50% of cases where only a solitary nodule is palpable, the goitre is actually multinodular with the other nodules simply being too small or indiscrete for palpation. Occasionally, a true solitary nodule can be due to adenoma, but it should never be attributed to this without exclusion of thyroid carcinoma.

Thyroid dysfunction

Goitre, thyroiditis, adenoma and carcinoma can all present with normal thyroid function (euthyroid), hyperthyroidism or hypothyroidism.

Hyperthyroidism

Hyperthyroidism is also termed thyrotoxicosis and is due to an excess of circulating thyroid hormone. Hyperthyroidism typically occurs in young women (Graves' disease), but also in patients with toxic multinodular goitre and hyperfunctioning nodules. Thyroid hormones increase the metabolic rate of all cells, the sensitivity of *beta*-adrenergic receptors and the growth of all cells (although this is mainly done by growth hormone).

Hyperthyroidism may manifest with a range of features:

- *General* – significant weight loss, heat intolerance, sweating and anxiety may occur.
- *Goitre* may be present.
- *Cardiovascular* – heart rate increases, arrhythmias such as atrial fibrillation may occur and the patient may notice palpitations. Hypertension may also occur. In extreme cases, cardiac failure may arise from the increased workload on the heart.
- *Gastrointestinal* – increased intestinal motility leads to diarrhoea.
- *Eyes*:
  - Lid lag (delay of lowering of the upper eyelid when looking down).
  - Graves' disease (see below) may also produce diplopia (double vision), lid retraction (retraction of the eyelids relative to the eyes) and exophthalmos (protrusion of the eye from the orbit). Pretibial myxoedema is also associated with Graves' disease; it appears as pink plaques on the anterior aspect of the lower leg.
- *Limbs* – a resting fine tremor and brisk muscle reflexes.

Graves' disease is the most common cause of hyperthyroidism. It is an autoimmune disease caused by immunoglobulin G (IgG) antibodies called long-acting thyroid stimulator (LATS) which activate the thyroid TSH receptor; it can be associated with other autoimmune diseases such as type I diabetes, pernicious anaemia and vitiligo. Graves' disease is treated by antithyroid drugs such as carbimazole or propyl-thiouracil, surgery (subtotal thyroidectomy) or radioactive iodine (I^{131}). Patients may become hypothyroid after treatment, especially after I^{131}.

Hypothyroidism

Hypothyroidism is also termed myxoedema and is due to a lack of circulating thyroid hormone, most commonly as an autoimmune phenomenon (atrophic hypothy-roidism). Hashimoto's thyroiditis (see thyroiditis section), thyroidectomy and iodine deficiency may also cause hypothyroidism. Drugs that may cause hypothyroidism include amiodarone (can also cause hyperthyroidism) and lithium.

The lack of thyroid hormone causes the reverse symptoms to those of hyperthy-roidism:

- *General* – reduced metabolic rate leads to lethargy, tiredness and decreased exercise tolerance. Depression is common. The voice is often coarse.
- *Goitre* may be present in iodine deficiency and Hashimoto's thyroiditis.
- *Cardiovascular* – bradycardia and hypotension may be present. Heart failure may be precipitated by this reduction in cardiac output.
- *Gastrointestinal* – decreased intestinal motility leads to constipation.

- *Musculoskeletal* – muscle reflexes are typically slow-relaxing, and a proximal myopathy may be evident.
- *Face* – classically, there is loss of the lateral third of the eyebrows, and a 'peaches and cream' complexion. Generalized hair loss may also occur.
- *Congenital hypothyroidism* – this is now an extremely rare disorder in the UK due to postnatal screening for hypothyroidism. Affected children have reduced intelligence and short stature.

Management is usually by thyroid replacement therapy, typically with oral thyroxine. If a sinister cause underlies the hypofunction, then thyroidectomy may be needed.

The 'sick euthyroid' patient

Thyroid function results may be spuriously abnormal in sick patients (e.g. with sepsis). This is because the peripheral conversion of T4 to T3 is reduced, there is a change in binding of serum proteins to circulating thyroid hormones and the level to TSH may be suppressed. In other words, *thyroid function tests are not reliable during periods of illness.*

Thyroid tumours

Thyroid tumours are commonly malignant (carcinoma or metastases) and only uncommonly benign (adenoma); it is rarely possible to distinguish the two before surgical excision. Primary thyroid neoplasms can be classified into:

1. Papillary carcinoma (the majority) – spreads via lymph, patients are usually euthyroid and it is often associated with prior radiation exposure.
2. Follicular carcinoma – spreads via the bloodstream and is generally more aggressive than the papillary type.
3. Medullary carcinoma – derived from the parafollicular C cells and spreads via lymph.
4. Anaplastic carcinoma – typically affects the elderly and is highly aggressive, with most patients dead within 1 year of diagnosis. Anaplastic tumours compress and invade local structures, causing dyspnoea (trachea), hoarseness of voice (recurrent laryngeal nerve), otalgia (vagus nerve), as well as giving rise to distant metastases (bone pain, pathological fractures) and systemic symptoms (malaise, weight loss).
5. Lymphoma (rare).

Total thyroidectomy is the mainstay of treatment for thyroid malignancies, with a few well-differentiated follicular carcinomas being treated with partial or hemithyroidectomy instead.

Metastases to the thyroid are uncommon and usually come from primary lesions of the breast, stomach, colon and lung.

Thyroiditis

- Subacute (de Quervain's) thyroiditis is caused by viral infection (e.g. Coxsackie, mumps). Notably, this painful condition produces low uptake on radioisotope scans. It is self-limiting and should resolve spontaneously.

- Postpartum thyroiditis may affect women up to 6 months after delivery. It also has low uptake on radioisotope scanning. It resolves spontaneously, but is strongly associated with hypothyroidism in later life.
- Hashimoto's thyroiditis may be associated with Graves' disease, etc. It produces a smooth non-tender goitre. Almost all cases are associated with antimyeloperoxidase antibodies. Only a minority of individuals are hypothyroid at their presentation with goitre. However, the remainder are at increased risk of future hypothyroidism.

Thyroidectomy

Complications include haemorrhage (which may cause airway obstruction and is an indication for surgical clip or suture removal followed by reoperation), hypothyroidism, recurrent laryngeal nerve damage (causing a change of voice), superior laryngeal nerve damage (causing a difficulty in voice projection) and inadvertent parathyroid gland removal (causing hypocalcaemia, typically presenting with carpopedal spasms). Thyroid crisis, a potentially fatal complication, is nowadays rare, due to careful preoperative preparation of hyperthyroid patients.

Dental aspects

1. The thyroid develops as a downgrowth from the foramen caecum at the junction of the posterior third with the anterior two-thirds of the tongue. Rarely, ectopic thyroid tissue remains in this tract and may be seen as a lump (lingual thyroid). This is often asymptomatic but may cause dysphagia, airway obstruction or even haemorrhage.
2. Patients with untreated hyperthyroidism can exhibit heightened anxiety and irritability. The sympathetic overactivity may lead to fainting.
3. Carbimazole occasionally causes agranulocytosis, which may cause oral ulceration.
4. The main danger in hypothyroid patients is of precipitating myxoedema coma by the use of sedatives (including diazepam), opioid analgesics (including codeine) or tranquillizers. These should therefore either be avoided or given in low dose.

Five facts

1. The thyroid gland uses iodine to synthesize the thyroid hormones thyroxine (tetra-iodo-thyronine, T4) and tri-iodo-thyronine (T3) which control the body's metabolic rate.
2. Goitre is an abnormal enlargement of the thyroid which, if large enough, may cause life-threatening upper airway obstruction.
3. A thyroid lump should be assumed to be cancer unless proven otherwise.
4. Sedatives (including diazepam), opioid analgesics (including codeine) or tranquillizers may precipitate myxoedema coma in hypothyroid patients, and thus should be avoided.
5. Ectopic thyroid tissue situated between the tongue and the thyroid gland may be seen as a 'lingual thyroid' lump, and can cause dysphagia, airway obstruction or even haemorrhage.

Transplantation

Each year, hundreds of thousands of patients are affected by life-threatening diseases which result in the need for transplantation. Transplantation is often the only effective treatment for end-stage disease.

Immunological principles

The major barrier to successful transplantation is immunological rejection of the transplant. The major histocompatibility region (MHC) or human leukocyte antigen (HLA) in humans is the main cause of immunological incompatibility. Located on chromosome 6, it consists of three classes, I, II and III.

HLA class I codes for HLA A, B and C genes, and HLA class I molecules are found on the surface of every nucleated cell in the body and function to present foreign, intracellular peptides to helper T cells, which in turn stimulate cytotoxic T cells to kill infected cells.

HLA class II codes for HLA DR, DQ and DP genes, and HLA class II molecules are found only on antigen-presenting cells (macrophages, dendritic cells) and present foreign, extracellular peptides to helper T cells, which in turn stimulate B cells to make antibodies against offending organisms.

HLA class III codes for TNF (tumour necrosis factor) and complement genes.

HLA classes I and II, particularly HLA B and DR matching, are the most important in organ transplantation. Rejection is best prevented by getting an exact match between the HLA of the host and the donor. However, except for transplants between identical twins, all transplant donors and recipients are immunologically incompatible to some degree. Serological and DNA methods are used for HLA typing.

Graft rejection

Rejection is the commonest cause of failure of organ transplantation. There are three types of rejection after organ transplantation:

1. Hyperacute rejection – due to preformed antibodies against graft HLA antigens (e.g. from blood transfusion, pregnancy or previous transplant).
2. Acute rejection – due to a T-cell mediated response (both helper and cytotoxic T cells are involved).
3. Chronic rejection – the mechanisms are less clear but are currently thought most likely to be T-cell mediated, possibly by a delayed-type hypersensitivity-type process.

All patients who have had a transplant in the past who feel unwell should be assessed promptly by a doctor, as early recognition and treatment of rejection is crucial. Immunosuppressive drugs such as ciclosporin, azathioprine, tacrolimus, sirolimus, mycophenolate and prednisolone are used. These not only suppress graft rejection but also cause T-cell immune defects and thus predispose recipients to viral, fungal and mycobacterial infections, and produce a liability after long-term use, to malignant disease, particularly lymphomas and, to a lesser extent, skin, cervical and lip cancer. Alternative anti-rejection agents acting on T cells, such as interleukin-2 receptor-blocking antibody preparations daclizumab and basiliximab, may avoid some of these complications.

Graft-versus-host disease is a rare, occasionally fatal, complication of HLA-mismatched grafting.

Renal transplantation

The kidney is the most common organ to be transplanted. A kidney from a living related donor or a cadaver is placed in one of the iliac fossae. The renal artery is anastomosed to the internal or external iliac artery, and the renal vein to the external iliac vein. The ureter is tunnelled into the bladder to prevent reflux.

The results of renal transplantation are improving, so that currently more than 80% of cadaveric kidneys are functioning at the end of 1 year. Renal transplant recipients now survive, on average, about 35 years. However, there is an extreme shortage of donor kidneys.

Other organs that are increasingly becoming transplanted are the heart, heart–lung, liver and pancreas. Bone marrow (haematopoietic stem cell) transplantation is increasingly used in the treatment of aplastic anaemia, leukaemias and other haematological malignancies, and some genetic defects.

Dental aspects

- Before transplantation there should be a full oral and dental evaluation and careful attention to oral and dental disease, bearing in mind that after transplantation the patient will be chronically immunosuppressed and at risk from infection.
- A full preventative oral health care programme should be instituted, and maintained at a high standard throughout and following transplantation.
- Oral candidosis may develop. The immunosuppressed patient is also prone to other oral infections such as herpes simplex or zoster, cytomegalovirus, Epstein–Barr virus, mycosis and toxoplasmosis. Rarely, oral or dental bacterial infections may spread, with serious complications.
- Drugs used in transplant patients, such as ciclosporin, nifedipine and basiliximab, may cause gingival swelling.
- Any invasive dental or drug treatment should only be carried out after consultation with the responsible physician and with due consideration to the bleeding tendency, any infectious risk and impaired drug metabolism. The responsible physician should be consulted with particular respect to the need for corticosteroid or antibiotic cover.

Five facts

1. Transplantation is the only effective treatment for many end-stage diseases.
2. The kidney is the most common organ to be transplanted.
3. Rejection is the commonest cause of failure of organ transplantation.
4. HLA matching is essential to prevent rejection.
5. Dental treatment after transplantation has an increased risk of infection and may require antibiotic and/or steroid cover.

Trauma and advanced trauma life support (ATLS)

Trauma is the commonest cause of death in 1–40 year olds in the UK. The distribution of trauma-related deaths is trimodal:

- 50% are 'immediate' (within seconds–minutes) and are due to primary central nervous system (CNS) injury or vascular lesions such as brainstem lacerations and aortic/large blood vessel lacerations.
- 30% are 'early' (minutes–hours) and are due to uncontrolled blood loss or secondary CNS damage. It is the 'early deaths' group in which intervention can prevent mortality, and as such this period is termed the 'golden hour'.
- 20% of trauma-related deaths are 'late' (days–weeks) and are caused by sepsis or multiple organ dysfunction syndrome (MODS).

In order to try to prevent morbidity and mortality in the 'golden hour', the American College of Surgeons developed the advanced trauma life support (ATLS) system, now used worldwide as an established method of trauma management.

ATLS is divided into primary survey, secondary survey and brief medical history. In this it differs from the standard order of history, examination, investigations and treatment that is the basis of all other medical work-ups.

Primary survey

The objective of the primary survey is to save life. Each of the following problems is dealt with chronologically:

A AIRWAY: check that the airway is patent and protect it. Ensure that the cervical spine is protected, especially in the unconscious or intoxicated patient with head or neck injuries.

B BREATHING: check that there is adequate, bilateral air entry and that there are no signs of life-threatening chest conditions (airway obstruction, tracheal disruption, open pneumothorax, massive haemothorax, flail chest and cardiac tamponade).

C CIRCULATION: detect shock and treat if present (see chapter on shock and haemorrhage). Obtain intravenous (IV) access using large-bore cannulae.

D DISABILITY: examine pupils for size, symmetry and response to light, and perform a brief neurological assessment using the 'AVPU' mnemonic:
    A = **A**lert
    V = Response to **V**erbal stimuli
    P = Response to **P**ainful stimuli
    U = **U**nresponsive

E EXPOSURE: completely undress the patient so as to inspect the entire body, including the spine.

Once the primary survey is completed, some basic investigations can be performed, such as a labstick glucose measurement (commonly referred to as a 'BM'), baseline blood tests, arterial blood gases, an electrocardiogram and the trauma panel of radiographs (chest, pelvis and possibly lateral cervical spine). After these, the trauma team progresses to the secondary survey.

Secondary survey

ABC is continually reassessed during the secondary survey, and if there is deterioration then the primary survey is restarted from the beginning. The objective of the secondary survey is to examine the patient thoroughly from head to toe, documenting injuries as they are found, so that they can be dealt with at the end of the survey.

The secondary survey includes performing a digital rectal examination, a vaginal examination in an adult female, otorhinoscopy and placement of a nasogastric tube (unless skull fracture suspected) and a urinary catheter (unless urethral injury suspected).

Medical history

If a medical history has not been taken while performing the primary and secondary surveys, then it is appropriate to take an AMPLE history at this point:

A = Allergies
M = Medications
P = Past medical history
L = Last meal
E = Events leading to injury

It is also important to check the patient's tetanus status and give prophylaxis if required.

Maintenance of airway

It is vital to be able to recognize a compromised airway (the single most important skill in the whole of medicine):

LOOK for facial/airway trauma, agitation, cyanosis and use of accessory muscles of ventilation.

LISTEN for stridor, gurgling, snoring or hoarseness.

FEEL for chest wall movement with ventilation.

Administer supplemental oxygen 15 L/min with a reservoir bag (do not waste time trying to find out if the patient has chronic obstructive pulmonary disease in case of carbon dioxide retention – hypoxia kills much quicker than hypercarbia in the trauma patient).

If the airway is obstructed, then clear any physical obstruction (teeth, foreign body or tongue), maintain the airway in an unobstructed position using a chin lift manoeuvre (the jaw thrust manoeuvre is contraindicated in trauma patients because of the risk of exacerbating cervical spine injury) and by inserting an oropharyngeal (Guedel) airway (a nasopharyngeal airway is an alternative except with facial trauma where brain injury may result with its use). It is important to reassess the airway after these initial attempts at securing it; if still inadequate, then a definitive airway is needed.

Definitive airways include orotracheal intubation, nasotracheal intubation and surgical airways (cricothyroidotomy and tracheostomy). These are best left to skilled anaesthetic personnel.

Maintenance of breathing

If ventilation is not adequate after the airway has been secured, ventilatory support may be needed. This can be delivered via mouth-to-mouth, mouth-to-mask, bag and mask or intermittent positive pressure ventilation (this may require paralysis and sedation of the patient by an anaesthetist).

Maintenance of circulation

Maintenance of circulation is dealt with in the chapter on shock and haemorrhage.

Dental aspects

- Maxillofacial injuries are common after road traffic accidents, and alcohol or other drugs are frequent cofactors. Assaults, industrial accidents, sport and epilepsy are other causes.
- Low-impact maxillofacial fractures rarely result in mortality if proper treatment is administered.
- High-impact maxillofacial fractures are often associated with other bodily injuries that may be life-threatening.
- Patients are often multiply injured and may have:
  - hazards to the airway
  - head injuries
  - damage to the cervical spine, thoracolumbar spine, eye, chest, liver, spleen, kidneys, long bones or bladder.
- Trauma to the maxillofacial area demands special attention since it may damage specialized functions, including breathing, seeing, hearing, smelling, eating and talking. Also, the vital structures in the head and neck region are intimately associated. The psychological impact of disfigurement can be devastating.
- Shock is most unusual in uncomplicated maxillofacial injuries or head injuries. Its presence is often an indication of internal haemorrhage.
- The possibility of pre-existing disease must always also be considered.
- The priorities of early management of a patient with maxillofacial and other injuries, especially if in coma, are:
  - Maintain a clear airway.

- Establish a neurological baseline from the history, consciousness level, examination and pupil reactions for future reference.
- Look for other serious injuries, in the thorax and abdomen, fractures of other bones, leakage of cerebrospinal fluid, and injuries to the eyes. The force necessary to create such severe maxillofacial injuries is usually significant enough to cause concomitant injury to the CNS, chest, abdomen, pelvis or extremities.
- Definitive treatment of a maxillofacial fracture must usually be delayed until the patient is out of danger.

- Because of the contiguity of the naso-oral passages and the perforating nature of these wounds, maxillofacial wounds are doubly exposed to bacterial contamination. The mouth, pharynx and nose are heavily populated by a variety of pathogens. All fractures in this region, except for fractures of the ascending ramus of the mandible, are compound and usually communicate with the internal mucous membrane wound and the external skin wound. Antibiotic therapy must begin early and be maintained.

Five facts

1. Trauma is the commonest cause of death in 1–40 year olds.
2. Airway (with cervical spine control), Breathing and Circulation (ABC) are the basic principles of ATLS.
3. Hypoxia kills first and must be dealt with before all else.
4. Constant reassessment of ABC is essential.
5. Maxillofacial injuries can damage specialized functions, including breathing, seeing, hearing, smelling, eating and talking.

Tuberculosis

Tuberculosis (TB) is an infectious disease caused by the bacterium *Mycobacterium tuberculosis*.

Epidemiology

TB is the most common serious infectious disease worldwide; approximately one-third of the world's population is infected. It is particularly common in the developing world.

The incidence of TB has been rising since the last decade due to the emergence of HIV co-infection and multi-drug-resistant TB (MDRTB) and it is increasingly encountered in the developed world, especially in patients infected with HIV. TB is now as common in London as in many parts of the developing world.

Pathology

Primary tuberculosis

Inhaled TB organisms migrate into the lung parenchyma and proliferate to form a primary site of infection called the Ghon focus. Infection then spreads to the draining hilar lymph nodes. The Ghon focus, together with surrounding infected lymph nodes, is referred to as the primary complex.

M. tuberculosis organisms are ingested by macrophages which are destroyed by a T-cell-mediated immune response, which leads to caseation (formation of pus) and necrosis. However, many TB organisms are able to survive in macrophages, and stimulate them to coalesce to form giant cells. These giant cells plus fibrosis surround a central area of caseation (like cheese) necrosis, the whole being termed a granuloma.

In most cases (90%), infection is self-limiting, but in a minority of cases infection may lead to progressive primary TB. Infection may then spread to the rest of the lung or into an adjacent bronchus or blood vessel. If organisms enter the bronchial tree, the patient becomes infective via respiratory spread; this is referred to as open or pulmonary TB. Blood-borne spread of organisms causes miliary TB.

Post-primary tuberculosis

In most cases, *M. tuberculosis* remains dormant in the primary complex. However, in a minority of cases, there may be reactivation. Exposure to further TB infection increases the chance of development of post-primary TB.

Susceptible individuals

Certain groups of individual are at increased risk of TB infection:

- immunocompromised patients, e.g. HIV infection/AIDS
- young children <2 years old
- *malnourished people*, e.g. alcoholics, homeless people.

Clinical features

TB is primarily associated with pulmonary disease; however, it is also associated with infection in a wide variety of organs.

Primary tuberculosis
The individual (usually a child) is usually asymptomatic, but may occasionally complain of a fever. Evidence of mediastinal lymphadenopathy (especially hilar) may be present on the chest radiograph. Other features include a unilateral pleural effusion and erythema nodosum (a tender rash over the shins).

Miliary tuberculosis
This disease is caused by severe and systemic TB infection. Marked constitutional symptoms of weight loss, tiredness and night sweats are present. Anaemia, leukopenia and hepatosplenomegaly are also common.

Post-primary tuberculosis
This disease (usually in adults) results in an illness characterized by fever (especially night sweats), weight loss, cough, shortness of breath and haemoptysis. Clinical features of lung lobe consolidation or collapse may be present. Cervical lymphadenopathy is non-tender. Lymph nodes may become fluctuant and discharge pus.

Although disease commonly remains confined to the lungs, extrapulmonary disease may occur (see below).

Extrapulmonary tuberculosis
Pericardial disease
Pericardial effusion and constrictive pericarditis may both result from TB. Hypotension, a raised jugulo-venous pressure and ascites may all be present. A pericardial effusion will produce a globular cardiac silhouette on chest radiography.

Gastrointestinal
Disease of the ileum and caecum is most common. Problems may include malabsorption, intestinal obstruction (from lymphadenopathy) or an abdominal mass (most commonly in the right iliac fossa).

Central nervous system
TB meningitis may present with headache, impaired consciousness, visual disturbance, vomiting or seizures. The course of disease is typically more chronic than that of acute bacterial meningitis.

Bone
Disease most often affects the spine (Pott's disease), where it may produce pain, fractures, cord compression or abscesses. This is a far commoner presentation in the developing world than in Western countries.

Diagnosis

Chest radiograph
A chest radiograph is the simplest screening tool for past or present TB. Scarring, consolidation or collapse, typically in the upper zones, should raise the suspicion of TB.

Sputum microscopy

Staining with either Ziehl–Nielsen or auramine is used to identify TB in sputum. Microscopy of other fluids (e.g. urine, cerebrospinal fluid) should be performed if extrapulmonary TB is suspected.

Culture

Culture using Lowenstein–Jensen medium is used to detect TB when microscopy is negative. TB is a difficult organism to culture; therefore it takes about 1 month for a definite result to be reached.

Bronchoscopy

Bronchoscopy may be used to obtain bronchial washings, which may be analysed with microscopy and culture.

Biopsy

Direct histological examination of tissue (lung, lymph node, bone, etc.) may lead to the identification of organisms.

Management

Chemotherapy

TB is difficult to eradicate, and requires combination chemotherapy over months. The recommended treatment regime is rifampicin, isoniazid, pyrazinamide and ethambutol for 2 months. After this, rifampicin and isoniazid should be continued for a further 4 months. MDRTB needs to be treated with 5 or more chemotherapy agents. There are significant side effects associated with combination therapy (Table 1).

Table 1 Major side effects associated with TB chemotherapy agents

Chemotherapy drug	Side effects
Rifampicin	Bodily secretions (e.g. tears, urine, saliva) become orange-stained
	Hepatitis
Isoniazid	Peripheral neuropathy
Pyrazinamide	Hepatitis
Ethambutol	Retinopathy

There is a high rate of non-compliance with chemotherapy for TB. This is explained largely by the long duration of chemotherapy and its significant side effects.

Directly observed therapy

The high rate of non-compliance with chemotherapy has led to the adoption of directly observed therapy (DOT) for selected patients. In DOT, patients attend hospital for each dose of their chemotherapy. It should be used in patients considered at high risk of not complying with treatment, e.g. alcoholics and psychiatric patients.

Vaccination

A national vaccination programme is vital to the prevention of TB in the population. In the UK, all school children are considered for vaccination.

The bacille Calmette-Guérin (BCG) vaccine is a live attenuated strain of *Mycobacterium bovis* which provides cross-immunity to TB. It is only given to individuals with a negative response to a tuberculin test. The Heaf test and Mantoux test are two types of tuberculin test which demonstrate an immune response to TB. A negative tuberculin test result is taken to indicate that no previous exposure to TB has occurred. A strongly positive tuberculin test result raises the possibility of TB infection, and should prompt further investigation as above.

Dental aspects

Pulmonary TB is of high infectivity. Dental treatment is thus best deferred until the infection has been treated. If patients with open pulmonary tuberculosis must be treated, special precautions should be used to prevent the release of mycobacteria into the air, to remove any that are present and to stop the inhalation by other persons. Reduction of splatter and aerosols, improved ventilation, ultraviolet germicidal light, masks, personal respirators and other personal protective devices, such as high-efficiency particulate air (HEPA) filters, are indicated.

TB occasionally presents with cervical lymph node enlargement, or oral ulcers or nodules.

Five facts

1. TB principally affects the lungs, and is caused by infection with the bacterium *Mycobacterium tuberculosis*.
2. The characteristic histological lesion of TB is the granuloma.
3. Initial infection with TB (primary TB) is often asymptomatic, but reactivation of disease (post primary TB) may occur several years later.
4. The treatment for pulmonary TB is quadruple therapy (rifampicin, isoniazid, pyrazinamide, ethambutol) for 2 months followed by rifampicin and isoniazid for a further 4 months.
5. Dental treatment is best deferred until TB has been treated, due to its high infectivity.

Upper respiratory tract infections

Upper respiratory tract infections (URTIs) are common illnesses, which range from benign conditions such as the common cold, to potentially life-threatening infections such as acute epiglottitis or influenza (the flu). Most URTIs are viral in aetiology (Table 1).

Table 1 URTIs and their main causative organisms

Condition	Microorganisms
Common cold	Coronavirus
	Coxsackie viruses
	ECHO viruses
	Parainfluenza virus
	Respiratory syncytial virus
	Rhinoviruses
Pharyngitis	Adenoviruses
	Coxsackie viruses
	Echoviruses
	Epstein–Barr virus
	Beta-haemolytic streptococci
	Influenza viruses
Tonsillitis	Adenoviruses
	Beta-haemolytic streptococci
	Enteroviruses
	Epstein–Barr virus
	Herpes simplex virus
	Influenza viruses
	Parainfluenza viruses
Influenza	Influenza viruses
Sinusitis	*Streptococcus pneumoniae*
	Haemophilus influenzae

Epidemiology

URTIs are especially prevalent in children, with the incidence highest during spring and autumn.

Spread tends to be in droplets via respiratory inhalation or the conjunctivae, or hand contact with infected surfaces, e.g. door handles. Spread occurs rapidly from person to person, which may lead to epidemics – especially with flu or the common cold.

Viral infections constantly mutate; therefore, immunity following infection does not lead to immunity for subsequent infections with the same virus. Thus, for example, an influenza pandemic may occur. The potential for this arises if the human influenza virus exchanges genetic material with an influenza virus that affects another species (most commonly a bird virus). The resultant virus is different to previously encountered viruses and therefore individuals have no immunity. Previous pandemics, although rare, have spread worldwide, leading to tens of millions of deaths.

Acute coryza (the common cold)

Coryza is extremely common and may be caused by a range of rhinoviruses such as adenovirus, coronavirus and respiratory syncytial virus. Features include rhinitis, causing an itchy nose, sneezing and clear or yellow nasal discharge of mucus. Pharyngitis may cause a sore throat and cough. Constitutional symptoms such as fever and lethargy are seen but, unlike in flu, myalgia and nausea/vomiting are absent. Illness is self-limiting to a few days.

Acute coryza may be complicated by secondary bacterial infection with *Staphylococcus aureus*, *Haemophilus influenzae* and/or *Streptococcus pneumoniae*, and can lead to sinusitis. Secretions then tend to be more purulent (yellow/green).

Lower respiratory tract infection such as laryngitis, bronchitis and pneumonia may result from direct spread of infection from the pharynx.

Sinusitis

The maxillary sinuses are especially susceptible to congestion of mucus due to poor drainage into the nasal cavity. This leads to facial pressure, pain and tenderness. Analgesia decongestants (e.g. ephedrine nose sprays) and antimicrobials may be needed.

Otitis media (infection of the middle ear)

Coryza blocks the Eustachian (nasopharygeal) tubes, impeding middle ear drainage of secretions and thus predisposing to infection. Pain and conductive hearing impairment are common. Antimicrobials may be indicated.

Acute laryngitis

Acute laryngitis causes a hoarse, painful voice, dry cough and a sore throat. The voice should be rested, together with analgesia and steam inhalation if necessary.

Investigation

Clinical evidence is sufficient for diagnosis of uncomplicated infection. An otoscope may be used to examine the middle ear. Change of colour and loss of the normal reflective pattern of light from the tympanic membrane indicates otitis media. A sinus radiograph may reveal loss of sinus radiolucency, which indicates congestion. A chest radiograph is needed if pneumonia is suspected.

Management

Acute coryza without complications is a benign and self-limiting condition. Simple measures such as rest and paracetamol (acetaminophen – to relieve fever and any pain) are sufficient. Antibiotics are not indicated.

Sinusitis, lower respiratory tract infection and otitis media, however, should be treated with antibiotics. Sinusitis is treated well with doxycycline. Otitis media may be treated with co-amoxiclav, in order to cover for *H. influenzae*. For treatment of lower respiratory tract infection, see the chapter on pneumonia.

Influenza

Influenza is caused by infection with either influenza A or B viruses but there are multiple strains. It starts as a URTI. Symptoms of rhinitis and pharygitis are very similar to those of acute coryza but, in addition, loss of appetite, nausea and vomiting, pyrexia and myalgia are also seen. Infection is usually acute and self-limiting but in the elderly or the immunosuppressed, complications, which may be severe or even fatal, may occur. Complications include secondary bacterial infection of the lower respiratory tract, tracheitis, bronchitis and pneumonia. Encephalitis and cardiomyopathy are rare.

Diagnosis of flu is clinical. Immunofluorescent and serological techniques are available to identify the causative virus, but this is only useful for monitoring of spread of flu in a population.

Treatment is conservative unless complications occur. Analgesics and antipyretics are used to relieve the symptoms. Aspirin must *never* be given to children under the age of 16 years who have flu-like symptoms, and particularly, fever. This can cause the rare but serious liver disease – Reye's syndrome. Antiviral treatment with zanamivir can shorten the time a person infected with influenza feels ill by approximately 1 day. Other antiviral drugs such as amantadine, rimantadine and oseltamivir may help but are reserved mainly for immunocompromised people, since these drugs can cause adverse effects.

Tonsillitis

The tonsils are areas of lymphoid tissue situated in the lateral wall of the oropharynx. They become inflamed during pharyngitis and become red, swollen and painful, causing a sore throat. Tonsillitis may also present with ear pain due to referred pain via the auriculotemporal branch of the facial nerve.

Most cases of tonsillitis are caused by viral infection (same organisms as coryza), but *Streptococcus pyogenes* may also cause tonsillitis. Treatment is usually conservative, but bacterial infections should be treated with amoxicillin. Occasionally, recurrent tonsillitis or persistently enlarged tonsils may require surgical excision (tonsillectomy). Generally, tonsillectomy is advised if the patient has >4 episodes of tonsillitis per year or >13 episodes in total. The most serious complication of tonsillitis and tonsillectomy is peritonsillar abscess (quinsy), which requires urgent surgery to avoid airway compromise.

Acute epiglottitis

Acute epiglottitis is a childhood infection with *H. influenzae* type B, which is potentially lethal, since epiglottic swelling may rapidly obstruct the airway; hence, it is a medical emergency. Acute epiglottitis presents with sore throat, breathlessness, stridor (inspiratory wheeze) and fever.

All cases must be sent immediately to hospital for paediatric assessment. Intravenous (IV) antibiotic therapy with co-amoxiclav should be started and, if necessary, endotracheal intubation should be performed by a senior anaesthetist. If endotracheal intubation proves impossible, a tracheostomy should be performed in order to relieve obstruction.

Under no circumstance should any attempt be made to examine the mouth or throat using a tongue depressor or any other instrument, since this may worsen any obstruction.

Croup (acute laryngotracheobronchitis)

The term croup refers to the abrupt onset of a barking cough, along with various combinations of stridor, hoarseness and/or respiratory distress. Initial symptoms consist of cough and sore throat. However, laryngeal involvement then occurs, which causes stridor and shortness of breath. Respiratory obstruction may be fatal without immediate treatment.

Croup is caused mainly by respiratory viruses, usually parainfluenza type 1, but also parainfluenza type 3, influenza A, adenovirus, respiratory syncytial virus, and echoviruses; *Mycoplasma* and other organisms may be implicated. As epiglottitis is an important differential diagnosis, immediate assessment by a hospital paediatric team must be sought. If necessary, endotracheal intubation or tracheostomy is performed to bypass the airways obstruction, but this is not usually needed. In the majority of cases the attack resolves after treatment with humidified air and oxygen, together with antibiotics (e.g. co-amoxiclav) and steroid nebulizers.

Dental aspects

1. Elective dental care is best deferred with the above conditions.
2. General anaesthesia should be avoided, since there is often some respiratory obstruction and infection can also be spread to the lungs.
3. Maxillary sinusitis can manifest with pain, which appears to emanate from the upper teeth.

Five facts

1. Most URTIs are viral in aetiology.
2. Complications of the common cold (acute coryza) include secondary bacterial infection, sinusitis, otitis media and acute laryngitis.
3. The most serious complication of tonsillitis and tonsillectomy is peritonsillar abscess (quinsy), which requires urgent surgery to avoid airway compromise.
4. If a child presents with acute stridor and breathlessness, refer for *immediate* paediatric assessment to exclude acute epiglottitis.
5. Do *not* attempt dental treatment or put any instrument inside the mouth if you suspect acute epiglottitis, since it may worsen upper airways obstruction and cause respiratory arrest.

Urinary tract infections

Urinary tract infection (UTI) is a broad term used to describe an inflammatory response of urothelium to an infectious agent. A UTI can involve either the upper urinary tract (kidneys) or the lower urinary tract (bladder and urethra). Pyelonephritis refers to a UTI involving the kidney and is characterized by fever, chills and flank pain. Cystitis is inflammation of the bladder and usually presents with dysuria (pain during micturition), frequency, urgency and suprapubic discomfort. This can be mistaken for urethritis in the female (see chapter on sexually transmitted diseases), but acute bacterial cystitis is much more common than primary urethritis in the female.

Classification

UTIs are termed either uncomplicated or complicated, by virtue of having underlying structural or functional abnormalities. *Uncomplicated* UTIs frequently arise in otherwise healthy adult females and usually respond well to antimicrobial treatment with few complications, but some women suffer from recurrent episodes. *Complicated* UTIs can be much more difficult to treat because an underlying abnormality such as calculi, diverticula, urinary obstruction, voiding dysfunction, congenital or post-surgical anatomical abnormalities, or long-term indwelling catheters can reduce the effectiveness of antimicrobial therapy.

Pathogenesis

Most UTIs in women arise from infections from the faecal reservoir ascending the short urethra from the vagina/perineum. The relatively long male urethra and its distance from the anus make this ascent more difficult in the male. Hence, any adult male presenting with a UTI should have full investigations to exclude structural and functional abnormalities (see later section). In women these investigations are deferred until typically the third episode of UTI.

It is now known that many women who suffer recurrent UTI but have no apparent underlying abnormality may have an increased adherence of bacteria to their vaginal and urethral surfaces and are more likely to have a nonsecretor blood group phenotype, suggesting that in others, secretory blood group antigens may have a protective effect.

Sexual intercourse significantly increases the risk of UTI in susceptible women. The vigorous activity of intercourse may cause urethral trauma, and probably 'milks' bacteria from the vagina or distal urethra up into the proximal urethra and bladder.

Aetiology

Most UTIs are caused by bacteria. In uncomplicated UTIs, *Escherichia coli* accounts for 80–90%, *Staphylococcus saprophyticus* 10–20%, and other Enterobacteriaceae such as *Klebsiella, Proteus* and *Enterobacter* account for the remaining uncomplicated UTIs. In complicated UTIs, Enterobacteriaceae are most prevalent. Gram-negative bacilli such as *Pseudomonas* and *Acinetobacter,* and Gram-positive organisms such as *Staphylococcus aureus* are also more common. *E. coli* accounts for only 20% of cases.

Bacterial cell surface structures called adhesins facilitate their binding to epithelial cell surface receptors. Certain adhesins contribute to bacterial virulence. The above pathogens are virulent in the urinary tract as they possess these adhesins.

Diagnosis

The diagnosis is usually based on the above clinical features. Urinalysis will show bacteriuria with pyuria (organisms and leukocytes in the urine), and a midstream urine sample (MSU) for culture should be carefully collected to reduce perineal contamination. It used to be stated that 100 000 colony-forming units (CFUs) had to be present for the diagnosis of UTI to be made, but it is now thought that as few as 100 CFUs/ml represents 'significant bacteriuria' in the symptomatic individual.

In most women presenting with uncomplicated UTIs, no additional investigations are required. Indications for urological work-up include haematuria, infection with urea-splitting bacteria, persistent breakthrough UTIs while on antimicrobial treatment, or any other reason for suspicion of a complicated UTI (e.g. history suggestive of calculus, prior urological surgery, male gender). In these cases, cystourethroscopy and upper urinary tract imaging (e.g. ultrasound), plus urodynamic investigation, voiding cystourethrography, retrograde ureteropyelography and renal scintigraphy may be indicated.

Treatment

Most uncomplicated UTIs respond well to a 3–5-day course of oral antimicrobials. Trimethoprim (TMP) is often used, but in some geographical areas UTIs are resistant to this and first-line therapy then consists of a quinolone such as ciprofloxacin. If symptoms persist, it is important to take a urine culture and adjust therapy based on the sensitivity results.

Recurrent uncomplicated UTIs are a difficult problem to overcome and most women are treated with a combination of hygienic advice regarding bladder emptying and perineal cleaning pre- and post-sexual intercourse, long-term low-dose antimicrobial prophylaxis (usually with TMP) and full-dose antimicrobial treatment when symptomatic. In cases of complicated UTI, it is vital to recognize and, if possible, treat these complicating factors. More powerful antimicrobial therapy (frequently quinolones) for longer durations (7–14 days) are indicated.

In cases of severe acute pyelonephritis, many patients require hospital admission for intravenous (IV) antimicrobials and hydration. In pregnancy, even asymptomatic bacteriuria should be treated, since the anatomical and physiological changes associated with pregnancy increase the risk of pyelonephritis, which, in turn, can lead to premature delivery and other complications.

Dental aspects

- UTIs usually have little relevance for dental care, although the symptoms may cause the patient to defer treatment.

- Cranberry (*Vaccinium macrocarpon*) juice, popularly used to prevent UTIs, may enhance warfarin activity.

Five facts

1. A UTI can involve either the upper urinary tract (kidneys) or the lower urinary tract (bladder and urethra).
2. Women are more prone to UTI than men, due to their urethras being shorter and close to the anus.
3. Any UTI in a man should be investigated for underlying structural abnormalities.
4. Recurrent UTI in women require investigation with ultrasound and cystoscopy.
5. Cranberry juice, often used to prevent UTI, can enhance warfarin activity.

Further reading

Standard medical and surgical texts, as in the list below, may be useful to the reader for more comprehensive information.

Browse NL. *An Introduction to the Symptoms and Signs of Surgical Disease.* 3rd Edn. Arnold: London, 1997.

Eaton DC, Pooler JP. *Vander's Renal Physiology.* 6th Edn. McGraw-Hill: New York, 2004.

Ellis H, Calne R, Watson C. *Lecture Notes on General Surgery.* 9th Edn. Blackwell Science: Oxford, 1998.

Gawkrodger DJ. *Dermatology – An Illustrated Colour Text.* 3rd Edn. Churchill Livingstone: Edinburgh, 2002.

Haslett C, Chilvers ER, Boon NA, et al (eds). *Davidson's Principles and Practice of Medicine.* 19th Edn. Churchill Livingstone: Edinburgh, 2002.

Hoffbrand AV, Pettit JE. *Essential Haematology.* 3rd Edn. Blackwell Science: Oxford, 1993.

Kingsnorth A, Majid A. *Principles of Surgical Practice.* Greenwich Medical Media: London, 2001.

Kirk RM, Mansfield AO, Cochrane PS. *Clinical Surgery in General.* 3rd Edn. Churchill Livingstone: Edinburgh, 1999.

Ramrakha PS, Moore KP. *Oxford Handbook of Acute Medicine.* Oxford University Press: Oxford, 1997.

Scully C, Cawson RA. *Medical Problems in Dentistry.* 5th Edn. Elsevier: Edinburgh and London, 2004.

Underwood M, Alexander R, Gurun M, Jones G. *Key Topics in Urology.* BIOS Scientific Publishers: Oxford, 2003.

Index